SAVED *and* HEALED

Receiving and Ministering
Divine Healing as Part of Salvation

DR. NNEKA O. IKE

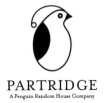

PARTRIDGE
A Penguin Random House Company

ISBN: Hardcover   978-1-4828-9042-6
            Softcover   978-1-4828-9043-3
            Ebook   978-1-4828-9044-0

To order additional copies of this book, contact
Toll Free 800 101 2657 (Singapore)
Toll Free 1 800 81 7340 (Malaysia)
orders.singapore@partridgepublishing.com

www.partridgepublishing.com/singapore

CONTENTS

Part two—Spiritual gifts

INTRODUCTION

T his book is divided into two parts. Part one is all about divine healing-how to receive and be able to also minister healing to others. Some of the stories in this book are real life stories without real names, while others are for illustration to drive home important points. There are questions for reflection at the end of each chapter in part one and the chapter on testimony. All questions for reflection are based on the content of this book and scriptural support. Personal testimonies, experiences and encounters with the Lord are encouraged during group discussions.

Part two is about spiritual gifts and biblical examples of the nine gifts of the Holy Spirit in operation.

God releases His saving and healing power through His word. **God sent forth His word and (it) healed them** (Psalm 107:20). **The gospel is the power of God unto salvation to everyone who believes** (Romans 1:16). The word of God works for whoever receives and acts on it by faith. **According to your faith will it be done unto you** (Matthew 9:29). However, God also touches and heals people out of His mercy and compassion. **Jesus saw the huge crowd as He stepped from the boat, and He had compassion on them and healed their sick** (Matthew 14:14). Having said that, it is very important to remember that as a believer in Jesus Christ, your faith in Him gives Him much pleasure. **And it is impossible to please God without faith . . .** (Hebrews 11:6).

Healing was included in Jesus' redemptive work. Your healing will be manifested eventually when you receive it by faith despite the symptoms or Doctor's reports. Receive healing by faith exactly as you received salvation by faith and believe that it is God's intentional will for you to be in good health. **But He was wounded**

for our transgressions, He was bruised for our iniquities; the chastisement for our peace was upon Him, by His stripes we are healed (Isaiah 53:5). **Beloved, I pray that you prosper in every way and (that your body) may keep well, even as (I know) your soul keeps well and prospers** (3 Jonh:2 Amp)

Satan is the source of sickness and disease. God gives life and health, satan brings sickness and death. Satan's primary agenda for you is to steal, kill and destroy everything good in your life. **The thief comes only to steal, kill and destroy; I have come that you may have life and have it to the full** (John 10:10). It is very important that you clear away any doubt in your mind that God wants you healthy even to your old age otherwise satan will rob you of one of your redemptive blessings. **I am the Lord who heals you** (Exodus 15:26b). **Even to your old age I am He and even to hair white with age will I carry you** (Isaiah 46:4). **Who satisfies your desires with good things so that your youth is renewed like the eagles** (Psalm 103:5)?

Jesus wants you alive and well so that you can join His mighty army on earth through your personal calling to preach the gospel of the kingdom of heaven, heal the sick and bring people to a personal knowledge of God through Him. **As you go, preach saying, The Kingdom of heaven is at hand! Cure the sick; raise the dead, drive out demons. Freely you have received, freely give** (Matthew 10:7&8). Satan's plan is to violently attack your mind, body and everything that you're blessed with to advance the kingdom of God. I am here to remind you that Jesus has given you all power and authority to violently take from satan and his demons everything about your life that is linked to the kingdom of God, especially your health. **And from the days of John the Baptist, the Kingdom of heaven has endured violent assault, and violent men seize if by force** (Matthew 11:12).

It was when the truths about God's will for all to be in good health and my restored authority over sickness and disease became real to me in regards to ministering divine healing to myself and to others that I decided to write this book.

This book is written in faith and confidence that any believer in Christ who reads it and ponders over the supporting Bible verses will not only receive healing, but will be inspired to go and boldly minister healing by the power of the Holy Spirit and in the name of Jesus to those who need it, just as Jesus did. **I assure you most solemnly I tell you, If anyone believes in me, he will himself do the things that I do; and he will do even greater things than these, because I go to the father.** (John 14:12).

No claim is made to have exhaustively written on the subject of divine healing. My main objective is to exhort every believer in Christ to rise and take their restored authority over satan, cast out demons, preach the Gospel and heal the sick as commanded by Jesus. **And when He had called His twelve disciples to Him, He gave them power over unclean spirits, to cast them out and to heal all kinds of sickness and all kinds of diseases.** (Matthew 10:1). This command has made it clear that no disease or sickness should be accepted by a believer in Christ as incurable. We have been commissioned and empowered by Jesus to **heal all kinds of sickness and all kinds of disease.** No exception.

ACKOWLEDGEMENTS

I am sincerely indebted to all my teachers in all the institutions of learning I trained in, whose spiritual insight and ideas have informed this book. I thank my lovely friend and husband, Henry Ike and our two beautiful daughters, Oge and Ogo for helping in creating and maintaining a loving and friendly home atmosphere that is conducive for growth and for writing this book.

Most importantly, thank you Holy Spirit for your help. Please bless everyone who reads this book, in Jesus' name. Amen.

DEDICATION

D edicated to my closest friend, the Holy Spirit; to the Ike's family; to the L.C. Efobi's family and to my global family, both known and yet to be known.

CHAPTER 1

WHERE IS SICKNESS FROM?

The answer to this question is obvious. Sickness is of course from satan. **Then satan went out from the presence of the Lord and struck Job with painful boils, from the sole of his feet to the crown of his head** (Job 2:7). **The thief comes only to steal, kill and destroy; I have come that they may have life, and have it to the full** (John 10:10). Satan is the thief and his primary objectives are to steal your health, kill you or destroy your spirit, body or mind by all means. It is unfortunate that somehow he has succeeded in convincing some people that God uses sickness and disease to either discipline or teach them some lessons. I used to think like that until I was finally delivered from self-righteousness through the message of the grace of Jesus Christ. Before then, I used to attribute every sickness or mishap I went through to God's displeasure of me or His discipline for my not being able to keep the laws in the Bible.

Todd asked, "Are you no longer keeping God's laws?" No Todd. Jesus did it all for me. He fulfilled everything God required of me from the law. **I have not come to abolish the law, but to fulfil it** (Matthew 5:1). **For if by one man's offense death reigned through the one, how much more those who receive abundance of grace and of the gift of righteousness will reign in life through the one, Jesus Christ.**(Romans 5:17 NKJV). As a result of God's righteousness on me, I no longer live by my own righteousness. **. . . and be found in Him, not having a righteousness of my own that comes from the law, but that which is through faith in Christ—the righteousness that comes from God is through faith** (Philippians 3:9).

1

Once I became secured in His righteousness that covers me, I began to see God differently. I began to see Him as a loving father who will not use sickness or disease to discipline me, just as I will not put sickness on any of my children as a means of discipline.

As my faith in Jesus grows, I personally experience the manifestation of the healing He obtained for me by His stripes as I lay hand on my body anytime the devil attacks it. **But He was wounded for our transgressions, He was bruised for our iniquities; the chastisement for our peace was upon Him, and by His stripes we are healed** (Isaiah 53:5). **And these signs will accomplish those who believe; in my name they will drive out demons; they will speak in new tongues; they will pick up serpents with their hands; and when they drink deadly poison, it will not hurt them at all; they will place their hands on sick people, and they will get well** (Mark 16: 17&18).

I am then totally convinced that being a loving father, God will never put sickness upon me for any reason and besides, He sent Jesus to take away sickness from me by His stripes. God will be negating what Jesus bore on my behalf by putting the same thing on me as a way of discipline or as a lesson. That will mean that Jesus' suffering for my punishment was for nothing. But it wasn't. His suffering brought me eternal salvation and healing. **Even though Jesus was God's Son, He learned obedience from things He suffered. In this way, God qualified Him as a perfect High Priest, and He became the source of eternal salvation for all those who obey Him.** (Hebrews 5:8&9). **He Himself bore our sins in His body on the tree so that we might die to sin and live for righteousness; by His wound you have been healed.** (1 Peter 2:24).

For you to receive healing from God, you also need to know and believe that He is the healer of all your diseases and not the bringer of them. Satan brings sickness, God heals. **Praise the Lord O my soul and forget not all His benefits—who forgives all your sins and heals all your diseases.** (Psalm 103:2&3). **For I am the Lord who heals you** (Exodus 15:26b). Believe that God meant it when He said He was the healer of His people during the Old Testament time. Believe that He is also your healer today. God is a covenant keeping God who kept His covenant of healing with His people as far as they diligently hearkened to the voice of their God and obeyed His commandments.

God's people believed His promise, obeyed His commands and the weak among them received strength and remained healthy and strong as their God led them out from Egypt toward their promised land. **He brought Israel forth also with silver and gold and there not one feeble person among their tribes** (Psalm 105:37). God extended His healing promise to you under a better covenant through your faith in what Jesus accomplished on the cross.

QUESTIONS FOR REFLECTION

1. What are satan's primary objectives?
2. From this chapter, it is obvious that sickness is from satan. What lies does he often tell to make people think otherwise?
3. On what would you base your faith for divine healing?

NOTES

CHAPTER 2

HEALING IS GOD'S WILL

Franca was a new Christian convert in her 30s and one of her favourite scriptures was the Lord's Prayer. She particularly loved the part that says . . . . **Your will be done on earth as it is in heaven.** (Matthew 6:9). Any time Franca was in doubt or uncertain about anything she was praying for, she would always say, "Lord, if it is your will, let me have this." Healing for her and her young children was always in her top list. She would always pray, "Lord, if it is your will, let my headache go, let Jessica's stomach ulcer go way, heal Joana's sore throat and let little Jonny's fever go away, amen."

What a list and what a wrong way to pray! No wonder why satan kept Franca and her family in bondage of perpetual sickness until she learnt the truth that healing for her and her children was and still is God's will, then they were set free. **And you will know the truth, and the truth shall make you free** (John: 32). **Teach me your ways, O Lord, that I may live according to your truth. Grant me purity of heart; so that I may honour you** (Psalm 86:11).

The truth remains that God wills that you live in good health. **Beloved, I wish above all things that you may prosper and be in health, even as your soul prospers** (3 John 2). **I will restore health to you, and will heal your wounds, says the Lord . . .** (Jeremiah 30:17). Jesus came to earth to do only the will of His father and by healing all that were sick, He demonstrated that it was God's will that people be healed and enjoy good health. **Jesus said to them, my food is to do the will of Him who sent me and to accomplish and completely finish His work.** (John 4:34). **Then I said, here I**

am, coming to do your will, O God (Hebrews 10:7). **The Son can do nothing by Himself. He does only what He sees the father doing, and in the same way** (John 5:19). Based on this truth, I believe that Jesus must have seen His father touching and healing the leper who said to Him, "If you are willing." **Then a leper came to Him, imploring Him, kneeling down to Him and saying to Him, "If you are willing, you can make me clean." And Jesus, moved with compassion, put out His hand and touched him and said to him, "I am willing; be cleansed." And at once, the leprosy left him and he was made clean** (Mark 1:40-42).

By his words, just like Franca's, the leper demonstrated an uncertainty and doubt about whether it was Jesus' will to heal him. Jesus nullified the leper's doubt expressed by the "if" by simply saying, "I am willing." In other words, God is willing. Your healing is absolutely God's will. Let this truth sink deep down and take root in your heart so that satan and his demons will no longer be able to tempt you to doubt God's will and desire to heal and keep you in good health.

Fred was a committed middle aged and sickly Christian man who served many years in his local Church. He was one of those Christians who did not grasp the biblical truths that **Christ redeemed us from the curse of the law** (Galatians 3:13) and that **Like a fluttering sparrow or a darting swallow, an undeserved curse will not land on it intended victim** (Proverbs 26:2). As a result, Fred lived all his life with sicknesses and diseases with the conviction that his family was cursed with asthma, allergy, cancer, diabetes and depression. Fred subconsciously owned every disease that had claimed the lives of his family members of previous generations. Though he allowed some fellow believers to lay hands and pray for him, he always cancelled their prayers with such statement as this, "Well I will eventually die of my cancer or diabetes because they run in my family." Unfortunately, Fred could not receive his healing and he died young of multiple sicknesses and diseases that wasted his body.

Our words express our convictions which are the unshakable beliefs that reside deep within us and which eventually create our outcomes. **Death and life are in the power of the tongue, and they who indulge in it shall eat the fruit of it** (Proverbs 18:21). **The good man from his inner good treasure flings forth good things, and the evil man out of his inner evil storehouse flings forth evil**

things (Matthew 12:35). We shall talk more on the importance of your words to your healing in another chapter, but for now, I encourage you to speak as your heavenly father speaks. He is . . . **the God who gives life to the dead and calls things that are not as though they were** (Roman 4: 17b). By speaking, God brought heaven and earth into existence. **In the beginning God created the heavens and the earth. Now the earth was formless and empty, darkness covers the surface of the deep and the Spirit of God was hovering over the waters. And God said, "Let there be light." and there was light** (Genesis 1:1-3).

Since God created you in His image and likeness, I submit to you that you were created to live and talk like Him. Use His words in the Bible concerning your healing and health and by faith call into existence your total healing. When satan points you to the symptoms, speak to him with the word of God as Jesus did. Say, satan, **It is written . . .** (Matt.4:4). **We live by faith, not by sight** (2 Corinthians 5:7). **But my righteous one will live by faith. And if he shrinks back, I will not be pleased with him. But we are not those who shrink back and are destroyed, but of those who believe and are saved** (Hebrews 10: 38&39). You already know that satan's main plan is to steal, kill and destroy you. To achieve his aim, he will always make you to focus your attention on the symptoms, the pain and all the negative reports to weaken your faith so he can destroy you. Do not let him. I remember one time I had a mouth injury from eating some tough food. My mouth was so sore that I couldn't open it wide or chew anything. I had to blend everything I ate. Though I had laid hand on myself and 'claimed' my healing, my daily practice was to go to the bathroom mirror and gaze at the injury for at least three minutes. One day, as I was 'fellowshipping' with the pain in the mirror, the Holy Spirit said, "Look unto Jesus and not the wound." I came to my senses, repented and fixed my eyes on Jesus as I spoke the word of God for healing over the injury. Glory to Jesus, I was totally healed the following day. It then made sense to me that whatever you focus on, you magnify. If you focus your attention on sickness and problems, you magnify them. If you focus on Jesus, He will be magnified. **Let us fix our eyes on Jesus, the author and finisher of our faith, who for the joy set before Him endure the cross, scorning its shame and sat down at the right hand of the throne of God.**

(Hebrews 12:2). **I look up to the mountains-does my help come from there? My help comes from the Lord who made heaven and earth** (Psalm 121:1&2).

QUESTIONS FOR REFLECTION

1. What type of prayer do some people pray that shows they doubt the willingness of God to heal the sick? How do you correct this mindset?
2. Who would you rather talk like to show your faith?
3. What is the best direction to turn in time of sickness or trouble and why?

NOTES

CHAPTER 3

IS GOD'S HEALING POWER EXCLUSIVELY FOR SOME?

J esus was one with His father when He was on earth and bowed His will to that of His father, doing nothing except what He saw Him doing. **I and the father are one** (John 10:30). **My father is always at work to this very day, and I, too am working** (John 5:17). **I tell you the truth, the Son can do nothing of Himself; He can only do what He sees His father doing because whatever the father does, the Son also does** (John 5:19). Where ever He went, Jesus healed all who were sick. **Great multitudes followed Him, and He healed them all.** (Matthew 12:15). **. . . and all who touched Him were healed** (Matthew 14:36b). **And all the multitude were seeking to touch Him, for healing power was all the while going forth from Him and curing them all** (Luke 6:19). We can see from the above Bible passages that the healing power of God was for all. By Jesus healing all who were sick and harassed by demons, He demonstrated that God delighted and still delights in healing and delivering anyone who is sick or is being oppressed by the devil.

Having been raised in a family where his father preferred his junior brother to him, Dennis, a 25-year-old Christian man believed that God has favourites when it comes to His dealings with people. This mindset has robbed Dennis of many blessings in the past, including healing and good health until he was radically set free from satan's lies during the preaching of the word of God in a youth conference. . . . . . **If you**

hold to my teaching you are really my disciples. Then you shall know the truth, and the truth will set you free (John 8:31&32). **My son, give attention to my words; incline your ear to my sayings, for they are life to those who find them, and health to all their flesh** (Proverbs 4:20&21). **He sent forth His word and healed them . . . .** (Psalm 107:20).

Not only was Dennis set free from the deceit of the devil through the preaching of the word of God, he has continued to renew his mind with the word of God. Dennis has finally come to realize that no one can be compared with God and that He does not have any favourites among His children like his earthly father does. **. . . I now realize how true it is that God does not show favouritism** (Act 10:34). **For the Lord your God is God of gods and Lord of lords, the great God, mighty and awesome, who shows no partiality and accepts no bribes** (Deut. 10: 17).

Today Dennis lives a victorious Christian life, in health and in the knowledge that Jesus provided healing for him and all mankind by His stripes. Besides, Dennis is now an effective witness to the young people he leads in his local Church. Some of the young people he leads are now operating in the gifts of the Holy Spirit, doing the works of Jesus. **I assure you, most solemnly I tell you, if anyone steadfastly believes in me, he will himself be able to do the things that I do; and he will do even greater things than these because I go to the father** (John 14:12). **And Jesus summoned to Him His twelve disciples and gave them power and authority over unclean spirits, to drive them out and cure all kinds of disease and all kinds of weakness and infirmity** (Matthew 10:1).

Until every Christian or even non—Christian understands the truth that God does not play favouritism but wants to heal every human being on earth, some redeemed people of God and others outside His Kingdom will still be bound by the lies of the devil that God wants to heal some and will not heal others. Again, until every believer in Jesus Christ is fully convinced that they can boldly minister the healing power of the Holy Spirit to the sick and operate in the gifts of the Holy Spirit as He leads, some Spirit filled believers will be bound by fear of failure or embarrassment. Geraldine said, "What if I lay my hands on the sick and they don't recover?" "I'll be so embarrassed." Well, Geraldine, if you believe in Jesus and you know that He cannot lie, then obey and lay your hands on the sick in the name of Jesus and leave the rest to Him. It is the Holy Spirit's job to manifest the healing Jesus paid for by His wound to those who need it. Just do as you are commanded. **And these signs will accompany those who believe ; in my name they will drive out demons; they will pick up snakes with their hands; and when they drink deadly poison, it will not hurt them at all; they will place hands on sick people, and they will get well** (Mark 16: 17). **When you enter a town and are welcomed, eat what is set before you. Heal the sick that are there and tell them, 'The kingdom of God is near you.'** (Luke 10:8&9).

The Command to heal the sick is for believers in Christ and it will be to every individual Christian according to their faith to minister healing to those who need it. On the other hand, God's divine healing is for all, whether they believe in Christ or not. God wants to heal all. If you need healing, believe that God wants to heal you. Open your heart and receive the manifestation of the healing that Jesus Christ has already made available by His stripes. God is inclusive and not exclusive.

If you are a believer in Jesus Christ, choose to step out of your comport zone, exercise your Christ given authority to cast out evil spirits and heal all kinds of disease. Don't worry and beat yourself up if it doesn't always turn out the way you anticipated. Be encouraged and keep believing the words of Jesus within you that the sick will recover as you lay your hands on them. You have a helper inside of you, the Holy Spirit who will help you to focus on Jesus instead of the outward appearances. **For I the Lord your God hold your right hand; I am the Lord, who say to you, fear not; I will help you!** (Isaiah 41:13). **Thus says the Lord who made you and formed you from the womb, who will help you; fear not, O Jacob, my servant and Jeshurun, whom I have chosen** (Isaiah 44:2). As a chosen vessel, lean entirely on the Holy Spirit with absolute trust and confidence in His power, wisdom and goodness and He will not fail to help you to do the works of Jesus. In victory over sickness, He will also help you to glorify Jesus so you don't take the credit.

QUESTIONS FOR REFLECTION

1. How can you prove that it is the will of God to heal all?
2. When will every spirit-filled believer in Christ rise and begin to boldly minister healing to the sick and operate in the gifts of the Holy Spirit as they are supposed to?
3. Explain in your words some of the greatest obstacles that prevent some believers in Christ from ministering healing to the sick. How can these obstacles be overcome?

NOTES

CHAPTER 4

WHOEVER BELIEVES

Have you ever wondered why so many people are not yet saved despite the fact that God loved and sent His Son Jesus to die so that no person in the world should perish in their sins? **God so loved the world, that He gave His only begotten Son, that whoever believes in him should not perish, but have everlasting life** (John 3:16). **The Lord is not slow in keeping His promise, as some understand slowness. He is patient with you, not wanting any to perish, but everyone to come to repentance** (2 Peter 3:9). The reason many are still not saved is because they have not obeyed, believed in Jesus Christ and surrendered their lives to Him through repentance.

Just as it is the will of God for all mankind to be saved, it is also His will for all to be healed and live in divine health. The redemptive work of Jesus included the saving of the human spirit from sin and the saving of human body and mind from sickness and disease. These two blessings were provided by the same Jesus, at the same time and by the blood that gushed out from His wounded body and so cannot be separated. Healing of the body and mind must then be received by the same faith by which salvation of the spirit is received. **But He was pierced for our transgressions, He was crushed for our iniquities; the punishment that brought us peace was upon Him, and by His wounds we are healed.** (Isaiah 53:5). **He Himself bore our sins in His body on the tree, so that we might die to sins and live for righteousness; by His wounds you have been healed** (1 Peter 2:24). **. . . . Anything is possible if a person believes** (Mark

9:23). **For it is by grace you have been saved, through faith—and this is not from yourselves, it is the gift of God—not by works, so that no one can boast** (Ephesians 2:8&9). . . . . **Believe in the Lord Jesus, and you will be saved—you and your household** (Acts 16:31). **Jesus said to him, "Receive your sight; your faith has healed you." Immediately he received his sight and followed Jesus . . .** (Luke 18:42). . . . . **Jesus said to the Centurion, "Go! It will be done just as you believed it would." And his servant was healed at that very hour** (Matthew 8:13).

Let this truth sink deep and take root in your heart that as you by faith have received the salvation of your spirit from sin, so shall you also receive by faith the manifestation of the healing of your body or mind which the stripes of Jesus provided for you.

Susan aged 16 said, "I am a Christian because my parents and my two big brothers are born again Christians and we all go to Church." No Susan, it doesn't work like that. You have to be born again by confessing, repenting of your sins and receiving Jesus into your heart before you can be saved and become a Christian. **Whoever believes and is baptised will be saved, but whoever does not believe will be condemned** (Mark 16:16). . . . . **Jesus declared, "I tell you the truth, no one can see the kingdom of God unless he is born again** (John 3: 3). Susan asked, "What does that mean?" Well, Susan, God made you through your Mum and Dad and you became their daughter. For you to be a Christian and a true daughter of God, the Holy Spirit has to join with your human spirit and give it a new birth, just as you were brought to this world by your natural parents. **Flesh gives birth to flesh, but the Spirit gives birth to spirit.** (John: 3: 6). **He saved us not because of the righteous things we have done, but because of His mercy. He washed away our sins, giving us a new birth and new life through the Holy Spirit** (Titus 3:5).

Just as the salvation of Susan's spirit depends entirely upon her personal faith and belief in Jesus, so also can she receive the manifestation of healing through her faith or through the faith of others. All through Jesus's earthly ministry, we also see Him healing people as a result of other people's faith. What mattered most to Jesus was faith in Him, whether it was the faith of the sick person or that of someone or some people laying hands on the sick or bringing them to Him, Jesus always responded to faith. **Some men came, bringing to**

Him a paralytic, carried by four of them. Since they could not get him to Jesus because of the crowd, they made an opening in the roof above Jesus and after digging through it, lowered the mat the paralysed man was lying on. When Jesus saw their faith, He said to the Paralytic, "Son, your sins are forgiven." . . . . He said to the paralytic, I tell you, get up, take your mat and go home." He got up, took his mat and walked out . . . . (Mark 2:3-5, 11&12a). **And these signs will accompany those who believe: in my name, they shall drive out demons . . . . they will place their hands on sick people, and they will get well** (Mark16:17&18).

Those who put their trust in Jesus, believe what He said and act on it are those who will confidently lay hands on the sick and have strong belief that the sick will receive their healing, whether instantly or progressively.

Claudia, a 45-year-old Christian woman, full of faith ran a small family fruit shop. One day, one of her lady customers in her 50s came complaining of a severe back pain caused by a slipped disc as diagnosed by her orthopaedic surgeon. Claudia said to her customer, "I know you don't follow my Christian faith, but my Jesus is willing to heal your back, would you let Him?" The lady said, "Okay." Claudia said, "I strongly believe that when I command your back to receive healing in the name of Jesus, It will." The lady nodded. Claudia stood beside the lady with her right hand at the woman's lower back. With a loud and authoritative voice, Claudia issued a command, "I command you slipped disc be in perfect alignment now in the name of Jesus. Pain leave this back in the name of Jesus."

When Claudia inquired, the lady said she was still in pain as before. Claudia knew that the healing power of Jesus was released by the Holy Spirit and that healing actually took place. She advised the lady to keep thanking Jesus. Well, I don't think that lady bothered to thank Jesus because she didn't see any reason to. But the following day she had every reason to praise Jesus because she was totally healed and had no need for surgery. When she excitedly brought the good news to Claudia, she received Jesus as her saviour and healer and joined Claudia's local Church.

There are countless real stories like this today where believers have stepped out and are still stepping out in faith, healing the sick, operating in the supernatural and bringing people to the kingdom of God as a result. As a believer in Christ, be convinced that Jesus meant it when He said that the sick would recover when you place your hands on them. Be bold and go for it in the name of Jesus. Ignore the symptoms and thank God for the sick person or persons to whom you have released healing. Let doubt, unbelief, fear and analytical reasoning go away in the name of Jesus. Amen!

QUESTIONS FOR RELECTION

1. Since it is the will of God that all be saved and healed, how must mankind receive these two fold blessings?
2. When is someone likely to receive healing through other people's faith?
3. What would you do if a sick person you laid your hands on and prayed for did not receive an instant healing? Give a personal example if possible.

NOTES

CHAPTER 5

SOME ARE HEALED AND SOME ARE NOT

D o you sometimes wonder why some people receive their healing and others don't despite the truth that God wants all to be healed? I am not claiming a straight answer to this question, but some things are definitely opposing God's divine will when some are healed and others are not. Sometimes it is ignorance of God's thoughts on sickness and disease that challenges the will of God so that some people live or die outside God's divine plan unless they know the truth that will set them free.

Sylvie, a 32-year—old Christian woman with a history of intermittent asthma since her teenage years was not taught at Church of her tradition that healing was included in the gospel of Jesus Christ. . . . . **and by His stripes we are healed** (Isaiah 53:5). **Everyone tried to touch Him, because healing power went out from Him, and He healed everyone** (Luke 6:19). In her early Christian days, Sylvie knew and memorised John 3:16—**For God so loved the world that He gave His only begotten Son, that whoever believes in Him shall not perish but have eternal life.** She has read Isaiah 53:5 her entire Christian life without knowing that she was already healed of her asthma by the stripes of Jesus, just as she was at the same time forgiven of all her sins by the same Jesus through the cross. This truth was not preached to Sylvie and so she lacked the faith that comes from the revealed word of God to receive the manifestation of her healing. . . . . **faith comes by hearing the message and the**

message is heard through the word of Christ (Romans 10:17). **My son, give attention to my words; incline your ear to my sayings, for they are life to those who find them, and health to all their flesh** (Proverbs 4:20, 22). Sylvie lived, thinking it was God's will to heal some and not heal others, and that she was one of those that would never be healed of that intermittent asthma. She was okay to suffer from the disease the rest of her life until she heard the good news about her healing for the first time from a visiting healing Evangelist. Sylvie testified, "Faith started to rise within me when the man of God stressed that sin and sickness had already been paid for through the suffering of Jesus and that everyone who believes, with no exception can receive forgiveness and healing at the same time." She continued, "As soon as he commanded healing for people suffering from asthma, I believed that my healing had come to me. I received it by faith and I noticed some heat in my chest and from that night asthma left my body forever to the glory of Jesus."

In order to fulfil Isaiah 53:5 and demonstrate that it is the will of God to heal all, Jesus healed all who were sick. **When evening had come, they brought Him many who were demon possessed. And He cast out the spirits with a word, and healed all who were sick, that it might be fulfilled which was spoken by Isaiah the prophet, saying: "He Himself took our infirmities and bore our sicknesses."** (Matthew 8:16&17). **Who Himself bore our sins in His body on the tree, that we, having died to sin, might live for righteousness; by whose stripes you were healed** (1 peter 2:24).

When the visiting Evangelist at Sylvie's local centre preached Jesus as saviour and healer, her faith rose and she received her healing. Peter presented Jesus as the healer to the cripple at the beautiful gate. **Then Peter said, "Silver and gold I do not have, but what I have I give you. In the name of Jesus of Nazareth, walk." Taking him by the right hand, he helped him up, and instantly the man's feet and ankles became strong. He jumped to his feet and began to walk . . .** (Acts 3: 6-8). Again, Peter preached Jesus as the healer to Aeneas. **"Aeneas,"** Peter said to him, **"Jesus Christ heals you. Get up and take care of your mat." Immediately Aeneas got up** (Acts 9:34). It is obvious in Acts 14:8-10 that Paul preached the good news of salvation from sin and sickness to raise the faith of a certain man at Lystra to receive healing. **And there sat a certain man at**

Lystra, impotent in his feet, being a cripple from his mother's womb, who never had walked: the same heard Paul speak: who steadfastly beholding him, and perceiving that he had faith to be healed, said with a loud voice, stand upright on your feet. And he leaped and walked.

More people will develop faith for healing if teachers and preachers of the gospel lay much emphasis on the truth that healing is part of the gospel of Jesus Christ and that it is for all as He demonstrated in His preaching and healing ministry. This is my encouragement-Whenever you preach Jesus, bring people's attention to the truth that He has already paid for their salvation and healing if they can believe. Make reference to salvation scriptures and healing scriptures, two of which are **For God loved the world that He gave His one and only Son, so that everyone who believes in Him will not perish but have eternal life** (John 3:16). **. . . by His stripes we are healed** (Isaiah 53:5), and others scriptures. By so doing, people's hearts can be prepared to receive from the Holy Spirit both the salvation of their spirits and the healing of their souls or bodies at the same time.

There are of course many other reasons why some people don't receive healing or minister healing, though God wants all mankind saved and healed. One of those reasons is unbelief which is sometimes caused by familiarity. **. . . A prophet is honoured everywhere except in his own hometown and among his relatives and his own family. And because of their unbelief, he couldn't do any miracles among them except to place his hands on a few sick people and heal them** (Mark 6:4&5). **. . . You faithless. How long will I be with you? . . . Bring the boy here to me. Then Jesus rebuked the demon in the boy, and it left him. From that moment the boy was well** (Matthew 17:17& 18).

QUESTIONS FOR REFLECTION

1. What in your own words prevents some people from receiving healing despite all prayers, while others do?
2. How did Jesus demonstrate that it was the will of God and still is the will of God to heal all with no exception?
3. What will make it easier for people to understand that healing is part of the gospel and consequently receive faith for it?

NOTES

CHAPTER 6

THE NAME OF JESUS

When God created man, He conferred honour to every human being so no matter what name any one is called by, they are still honoured and blessed by God in different ways. **What is man that you are mindful of him, the son of man that you care for him? You made him a little lower than the heavenly beings and crowned him with glory and honour. You made him ruler over the works of your hands and put everything under his feet** (Psalm 8:4-6). **Since you are precious and honoured in my sight, and because I love you, I will give men in exchange for you, and people in exchange for your life** (Isaiah 43: 4).

Jesus satisfied His father by dying to redeem the honour that God bestowed to man before man sinned. Having accomplished that through the cross, He inherited a name above every name, the name that everything must bow to, including sicknesses, diseases and infirmities. **And being found in appearance as a man, he humbled himself and became obedient to death and even death on a cross. Therefore God exalted Him to the highest place and gave Him the name above every name, that at the name of Jesus every knee should bow in heaven and on earth and under the earth, and every tongue confess that Jesus Christ is Lord to the glory of God the father** (Philippians 2:8-11). **Then Jesus came and spoke to them saying, "All authority has been given to me in heaven and on earth."** (Matthew 28:19).

The Omnipotence of God dwells in the Name of Jesus so much that Jesus charged His believers to go and do exploit in His name. . . . ."**Go into all the world and preach the gospel to every creature . . . ." And these signs shall follow those who believe: in my name they will cast out demons; they will speak with new tongues; they will take up serpents; and if they drink anything deadly, it will by no means hurt them; they will lay hands on the sick, and they will recover** (Mark 16:17&18). **You did not choose me, but I chose you and appointed you that you should go and bear fruit, and that your fruit should remain, that whatever you ask the father in my name He may give you** (John 15:16).

You are chosen and commissioned by Jesus to preach the gospel to the lost, heal the sick and bear fruit that will remain, including sons and daughters that will remain in the Kingdom of God. Note that you are representing the enthroned Jesus when you boldly use His name and His authority to heal the sick and do even greater works than He did.

When, by faith you command demons and sickness to go in the name of Jesus, they must bow and go because it is like Jesus Himself issuing the command. **The seventy two returned with Joy and said, "Lord, even the demons submit to us in your name." He replied, "I saw satan fall like lightning from heaven. I have given you authority to trample on snakes and scorpions and to overcome all the power of the enemy; nothing will harm you."** (Luke 10:17-19). **Then Philip went down to the city of Samaria and preached Christ to them. And the multitudes with one accord heeded the things spoken by Philip, hearing and seeing the miracles which he did. For unclean spirits, crying with a loud voice came out of many who were possessed; and many who were paralysed and lame were healed . . . .** (Acts 8:5-8).

Sally, a 35-year Christian woman said, "I doubt if the Lord will ever use me the way He used Philip or the way He is using today's well known Evangelists." Well, Sally, the Lord wants to use you in the area He has called you. However, whichever area you are called, Jesus wants you to be His witness. That is why He baptises His believers in the Holy Spirit, so that we can, through words and deeds be His witnesses. **"You shall receive power when the Holy Spirit has come upon you; and you shall be witnesses to me in Jerusalem, and in all Judea and Samaria, and to the end of the earth**(Acts 1:8). **I assure you, most solemnly I tell you, if anyone steadfastly believes in** me, he will himself be able to do the things that I do; and he will do even greater things than these, because I go to the father ((John 14:12).

If Sally believes in Jesus and has been baptised in the Holy Spirit, she can by His power do all the works that Jesus did. For example, Jesus taught, He preached, He healed all kinds sicknesses besides casting out demons, raising the dead and setting the captives free. **The Spirit of the Lord is upon me, for He has anointed me to bring Good News to the poor. He has sent me to proclaim that captives will be released, that the blind will see, that the oppressed will be set free, and that the time of the Lord's favour has come** (Luke 4:18). **Jesus went about all the cities and villages, teaching in their Synagogues, preaching the gospel of the kingdom, and healing every disease among the people** (Matthew 9:35). Every believer in Christ is qualified to do the work of Jesus. Only faith in the Holy Spirit, boldness and the name of Jesus are required. Philip, who was like today's Church volunteer, not even among the twelve disciples, stepped out in faith like the apostles and preached Christ and the Lord confirmed what he said with healing miracles. **Many evil spirits were cast out . . . . and many who had been paralysed or lame were healed. So there was great joy in that city** (Acts 8: 7&8). **And the disciples went everywhere and preached, and the Lord worked through them, confirming what they said by many miraculous signs** (Mark 16:20).

QUESTIONS FOR REFLECTION
1. What is in the name of Jesus? Explain.
2. How do you represent the enthroned king Jesus in the great commission?
3. What is the main reason for the baptism in the Holy Spirit?

NOTES

CHAPTER 7

PRAYER OF AGREEMENT IS EFFECTIVE

When believers in Christ stand together in agreement and command healing in the name of Jesus for a non-believer in Christ or even for a believer who is so sick to use their own faith, healing will occur because they unite their faith and God honours faith . . . **I tell you the truth, if you have faith and don't doubt, . . . you can say to this mountain, 'may you be lifted up and thrown into the sea' and it will happen** (Matthew 21:21). **If two of you shall agree on earth as touching anything that they shall ask, it shall be done for them by my father who is in heaven. Where two or three are gathered together in my name, I am there in the midst of them** (Matthew 18:19-20). **One day peter and John were going up to the temple . . . . Now a man crippled was being carried to the temple gate called Beautiful where He was put every day to beg . . . . When he saw Peter and John about to enter, He asked them for money. Peter looked straight at him, as did John. Then Peter said, "Silver or gold I do not have, but what I have I give you. In the name of Jesus Christ of Nazareth, walk." Taking him by the right hand, he helped him up, and immediately the man's feet and ankles became strong. He jumped to his feet and began to walk** (Acts 3:1-8). Notice in verse 4 that Peter looked straight at the crippled man as John did. That suggests that both apostles agreed that what the man needed was healing and not money. Their agreement on the need of the crippled man and their united faith in the name of Jesus restored health to the sick.

Darren, a 51-year old man was experiencing severe pain in his bowel and an unclear diagnosis suggested it could be bowel cancer. No sooner had Darren heard the report than he was seized with an intense fear until some Church leaders who just came for a social visit heard about his condition and prayed for him in agreement. When he went for the result of the previous tests, Darren was cleared of any cancer and he is totally well till date to the glory of Jesus.

Joana asked," What if the sick person does not believe, will he or she still be healed through the agreement of those who believe?" Joana, God is a gracious God and does not deal with us according to our sins.Yes sometimes out of His mercy, He ignores human weakness like the unbelief and doubt of the sick or afflicted person and heals them through the faith of those who agree on their behalf. For example, One Shunammite woman did not believe she could conceive a Child in her condition and her husband's old age. She was healed of bareness anyway, in spite of her unbelief. **Later Elisha said, what then is to be done for her? Gahazi** (Elisha's servant) **answered, she has no child and her husband is old. He said, call her. Gehazi called her . . . . Elisha said, at this season when the time comes around, you shall embrace a son. She said, no, my lord, you man of God, do not lie to your handmaid. But the woman conceived and bore a son at that season . . .** (2 Kings 4:14-17). **Jesus saw the huge crowd as He stepped from the boat, and He had compassion on them and healed their sick** (Matthew 14:14).

Other than God's demonstration of His love in healing those who do not believe, you can please God only through faith. **And without faith it is impossible to please God, because anyone who comes to Him must believe that He exists and that He rewards those who earnestly seek Him** (Hebrews11:6). **As Jesus went on from there, two blind men followed him, calling out, "Have mercy on us, Son of David" . . . . He asked them, "Do you believe that I am able to do this?" "Yes Lord" they replied. Then He touched their eyes and said, "According to your faith, let it be done to you." And their sight was restored . . . (Matthew 9:29-30).**

QUESTIONS FOR REFLECTION

1. What makes prayer of agreement effective? Explain
2. What motivates God to heal even those who do not believe?
3. What pleases God the most?

NOTES

CHAPTER 8

ANOINTING THE SICK WITH OIL

il in the Bible is one of the symbols of the Holy Spirit that indicates not only His enabling but also His healing power. **How God anointed Jesus of Nazareth with the Holy Ghost and with power; who went about doing good, and healing all that were oppressed of the devil; for God was with Him**. (Acts 10:38). **And they cast out many demons and healed many sick people, anointing them with olive oil** (Mark 6:13). **Is any sick among you? Call for the elders of the Church; and let them pray over the sick, anointing them with oil in the name of the Lord. The prayer of faith shall save the sick, and the Lord shall raise them up; and if they have committed sins, they shall be forgiven** (James 5:14). It is not the elders or the oil that heals, but the Holy Spirit who releases His healing power into the body of the sick. It is then imperative that the elders put their total faith in the Holy Spirit as they anoint the sick with oil and pray for the sick so that He will raise them up.

No matter how hopeless the situation is, no matter what the doctor's report is, and no matter how 'incurable' the sickness has been labelled, the elders of the Church should bear in mind that it is the will of God to heal the sick they are anointing with oil and praying for, and that He doesn't want them to die of that disease. The Holy Spirit in His mercy will release the gift of faith to anyone who has such mindset with which they will believe the impossible and minister healing to the sick in different ways, including anointing them with oil.

When you are being prayed for, release your faith if you are physically, mentally and emotionally able to. Believe that God wants you totally healed. This is good news that should lift your spirit to believe the Holy Spirit to transmit His healing power from the anointing oil to your body. This is vital, especially if you have previously believed that healing is just for some people and not for others or worse still, that there is limit to what sickness God could heal.

Magda, a Christian Minister in her late 40s was diagnosed with an aggressive form of breast cancer, but despite the bad report and even the failing faith of those around her, she stood firm on her faith in Jesus and on His finished work for her. No day passed without Magda confessing all the healing scriptures inspired by the Holy Spirit and believing that she was already healed since she had cried unto God to save her body from cancer. **When Jesus had received the sour wine, He said it is finished! And He bowed His head and gave up His Spirit** (John 19:30). **O Lord my God, I cried to you and you have healed me. O Lord, you have brought my life up from Sheol (the place of the dead); you have kept me alive, that I should not go down to the pit (the grave).** (Psalm 30:2-3 AMP.) Glory to God that Jesus miraculously and totally healed Magda of breast cancer according to her faith.

It is **the prayer of faith that shall save the sick** (James 5:15) as the elders of the Church anoint the sick with oil. Faith is released into the spirit man through the word of God. **And take the helmet of salvation, and sword of the Spirit, which is the word of God. Praying always with all prayer and supplication . . .** (Ephesians 6:17, 18a). **Let the saints rejoice in this honour and sing for joy on their beds. May the praise of God be in their mouth and a double-edge sword in their hands to afflict vengeance on the nations and punishment on the peoples, to bind their kings with fetters, and their nobles with shackles of iron, to carry out the sentence written against them. This is the glory of all His saints. Praise the Lord.** (Psalm 149:5-9).

When you have an unshakeable faith and confidence that there is nothing in the mind of God that wishes you sickness after He sent Jesus to take those painful lashes on His body and healed you by His stripes, then you can stand tall in your inner man like Magda did and receive your healing no matter what people think or don't think. God has made it absolutely clear in the Scriptures that it is His will for you to live in good health and receive healing from any type of sickness. . . . **I am the Lord who heals you** (Exodus 15:26). **Praise the Lord o my soul . . . . who heals all your diseases** (Psalm 103:3). **. . . . by His stripes we are healed** (Isaiah 53:5). **. . . . I will take away sickness from among you** (Exodus 23:25). Even if your time on earth is finished or you are in your old age, God wants you well first, then He can go ahead and take your breath. **Abraham lived 175 years and he died at a ripe old age, having lived a long and satisfying life** (Genesis 25:7&8). **Moses was 120 years old when he died, yet his eyesight was clear, he was as strong as ever** (Deuteronomy: 34:7). If you believe it shall be so for you. Say a big AMEN and it shall be to you as you have believed. **Then Jesus said to the Centurion, Go! It will be done just as you believed it would. And his servant was healed at that very hour** (Matthew 8:13). **. . . . Jesus said, everything is possible for him who believes.** (Mark 9: 23). Jesus said, **everything** and not **some things** are possible if you can dare to believe Him. Don't limit God because He will never withhold from you anything that will bring Him glory, including your healing and divine health all through your life, if you believe.

QUESTIONS FOR REFLECTION
1. Oil is one of the symbols of the Holy Spirit. Explain.
2. What would be uppermost in your heart as you anoint the sick with oil?
3. What will help you as a believer in Christ to stand firm and receive healing despite medical reports and perhaps the failing faith of those around you?

NOTES

CHAPTER 9

GOD'S HEALING POWER THROUGH HANDS

Here is one of the declarations our children make after every family devotion—*"Accountability."* (Usually said by either parent) and the children's response is—*"Responsibility." "You do your part, I do my part."* The rationale behind this declaration is to remind ourselves that each person has the responsibility of playing his or her own role in maintaining the smooth running of our family and that we are all accountable to each other. I wish I could tell you that it's always the case, but in most cases, the principle has been working for us.

The same principle is applicable to Jesus' commission to all believers in Him to minister healing to the sick by laying on of hands. **These signs shall follow them that believe: in my name they shall cast out devils; they shall lay hands on the sick, and they shall recover** (Mark 16:17). In almost all cases, for the will of God to be accomplished on earth, there is usually man's part and God's part. The believer in Christ has to lay hands on the sick then the Holy Spirit will cause them to recover.

Veronica asked, "As a believer in Christ, do I always have to lay hands on the sick before they recover?" There are many ways of ministering healing to the sick Veronica, however laying on of hands is one of the most common ways of ministering healing especially if the sick is within a close range. By laying your hands on the sick, you have become a direct contact through which God's healing power is transmitted to another person. **The father of Publius lay sick of a fever and of a bloody flux: Paul went in and prayed, and laid his hands on him, and healed him.** (Acts 28:8). **Then one of the synagogue rulers named Jairus, came there. Seeing Jesus, he fell at His feet and pleaded earnestly with Him, "My little daughter is dying. Please come and put your hands on her so that she will be healed and live." . . . . Jesus told the synagogue leader, "Don't be afraid; just believe . . . . He took her by the hand and said, "Talitha Koum!" which means, "Little girl I say to you get up!" Immediately the girl got up and walked around.** (Mark 5:22, 30 and 41). The resurrection power of the Holy Spirit was transmitted from Jesus' hand to the dead little girl and she came alive.

If you are a believer in Christ filled with the Holy Spirit, you have the nature and power of God in you. The word 'power' is the Greek word *"dunamis"* from which the English word "dynamite" was derived and it connotes explosive power in Greek language. *Dunamis* is the descriptive word for God's explosive power which was at work in Jesus when He was on earth. The apostles demonstrated this mighty power of God and it is the same power that every believer receives when they are baptised in the Holy Spirit. This power of God within us as believers in Christ is immeasurable and unlimited. All we need is a revelation of the mighty power within us so we can demonstrate it to the world by healing all kinds of diseases and be effective witnesses of Jesus Christ in many ways. **But you shall receive power when the Holy Spirit comes on you; and you will be my witnesses in Jerusalem, and in all Judea and Samaria, and to the ends of the earth** (Acts 1:8). **And (so you can know and understand) what is the immeasurable and unlimited and surpassing greatness of His power in and for us who believe, as demonstrated in the working of His mighty strength** (Ephesians 1:19. AMP). This mighty power, the presence of God or His glory can flow through your hands if you are a believer in Jesus Christ to heal the sick and they shall recover, Jesus assured. This should be your expectation. No thinking twice about it, whether or not it will work. Just do what you are commissioned to do as He leads you and the Holy Spirit will manifest the healing that Jesus' wounds had already secured for the sick.

If you are sick and you let a believer or believers in Jesus Christ to lay hands on you, your part is just to believe like little Johnny whose mother promised to buy him an Air Plane. He simply believed her mother's promise. All day long while his mother was at the shopping mall, Jonny was full of expectation. He couldn't wait to fly his Air Plane. No sooner had mother arrived than Johnny happily skipped to her and the first shopping bag he grabbed was the one that had his toy Air plane. Johnny pulled it out and off he went to the front yard to fly to wherever he had scheduled to 'fly' to. Little Johnny was happy with his toy Air Plane, not caring about the ones that might be arriving or departing any of the world's Air Ports.

Jesus wants us to receive everything He died to give us (I call them kingdom blessings, which include divine healing) like little Johnny, living by faith and trusting Him. **I tell you the truth, anyone who will not receive the kingdom of God like a little child will never enter it** (Luke 18:17). **When He has gone indoors, the blind men came to Him, and He asked them, "Do you believe I can do this?" "Yes Lord" they replied. Then He touched their eyes and said, "According to your faith will it be done to you" and their sight was restored to them . . .** (Matthew 9:28-30). Robin said, "I didn't feel anything when some Christians came over and laid hands on me." Yes, Robin, sometimes sick people don't feel anything when believers in Christ lay hands on them, but that doesn't mean that healing has not taken place. Christian faith is not based on feelings or on outward appearances, but by what the word of God says. In some cases, healing is accompanied by some sensations, heat or vibration while at other times it is not. Sometimes healing is instant, at other times it is progressive. Whichever way, just believe.

QUESTIONS FOR REFLECTION

1. As a Spirit filled believer, what type of power is transmitted from you to the body of the sick person on whom you lay your hands? Explain.
2. Do you have confidence that when you lay your hands on the sick they will recover? If yes, where does the confidence come from? If no, share your thoughts.
3. When you need divine healing as part of kingdom blessing, what type of faith does Jesus advocate?

NOTES

CHAPTER 10

SALVATION AND HEALING

When you know the truth that healing is part of the redemptive work which Jesus accomplished for you on the cross, you see yourself already healed when you fall sick despite the symptoms, just as you see yourself already saved despite your failings or shortcomings. For you to walk in victory over sickness and disease, you have to give thanks to God both in health and in sickness for the healing Jesus obtained for you.

Tell your soul like David did when he said, **Praise the Lord O my soul, and forget not all His benefits-who forgives all your sins and heals all your diseases** (Psalm 103:2&3). **Who His own self bore our sins in His own body on the tree, that we, being dead to sins should live in righteousness; by whose stripes we are healed** (1 Peter 2:24). The devil thrives in the ignorance or the forgetfulness of the believer of his or her inheritance, their authority over the powers of darkness and diseases through the cross. He is happy when you don't often think of Jesus as your substitute who was made sick and sinful for you; who took every one of your sins and sickness upon Himself so you don't have to suffer. Satan knows that he has no legal right to lay on you again what Jesus took away from you, so he makes you forget what the cross was all about and directs your focus on the symptoms so you don't look to Jesus. **We live by faith not by sight** (2 Corinthians 5:7). **Let us fix our eyes on Jesus, the author and finisher of our faith, who for the joy set before Him endured the cross, scorning its shame and sat down at the right hand of the throne of God** (Hebrews 12:2).

Mrs Francis is a 55-old Christian woman who suffered from a debilitating form of rheumatoid arthritis for nearly a decade. Before her total healing during a miracle service, Mrs Francis, originally from a non-charismatic Christian background, though born again, was not taught the truth that healing for her body was part of Jesus' redemptive work as emphatically and positively as the truth about her spiritual salvation was instilled into her at her new birth. Consequently, Mrs Francis lived with sickness for nearly ten years not believing for healing in the same way she has believed in her secured forgiveness of all her sins; the righteousness of God that covers her and her eternal life with God through Jesus. As long as Mrs Francis was not fully sure that God wanted and still wants her to be well, she always doubted as to whether or not she would be healed. She received an instant healing when the good news of healing was preached in a miracle service. The word of God produced faith in her heart for healing. **Consequently, faith comes from hearing the message, and the message is heard through the word of Christ** (Romans 10:17). **I am not ashamed of the gospel because it is the power of God for the salvation of everyone who believes: first for the Jew, then for the Gentile** (Romans 1:16).

Jesus suffered and secured the salvation of the spirit as well as that of the body and mind and this good news should be preached all through the world otherwise people will not develop faith to receive the healing that has already been made available by Jesus. **But He was pierced for our transgressions, He was crushed for our iniquities; the punishment that brought us peace was upon Him, and by His wounds we are healed** (Isaiah 53:5). **He said to them, "Go into all the world and preach the good to all creature** (Mark 16:15). **He called His twelve disciples to Him and gave them authority to drive out evil spirits and to heal every disease and sickness** (Matthew 10:1).

All through the books of Matthew, Mark, Luke and John in the Holy Bible, you will see Jesus, preaching the good news, teaching, healing the sick and casting out demons from people. Bringing relief to mankind of their physical as well as spiritual problems was a significant part of Jesus' earthly ministry. Jesus' healing ministry was a direct expression of God's will to heal all. In regards to the man born blind, Jesus said to His disciples, **As long as it is day, we must do** the work of Him who sent me. Night is coming when no one can work (John 9.4). To John the Baptist's disciples, Jesus said, **Go and tell John what you hear and see: the blind receive their sight and the lame walk, lepers are cleansed and the deaf hear, and the dead are raised up, and the poor have good news preached to them** (Mark 11:3-11).

QUESTIONS FOR REFLECTION
1. How did God provide salvation and healing? How are they to be received? Explain.
2. Why is it important to emphasise divine healing as part of the redemptive work of Jesus when you preach the gospel?
3. How did Jesus demonstrate God's will to heal all?

NOTES

CHAPTER 11

RECEIVING AND MINISTERING DIVINE HEALING AS PART OF SALVATION

Everything you go through in life, every battle you win by the grace of God and every blessing you receive from God is for the benefit of another person. You receive so you can give what you have. Once you have the conviction that God wants you and other human beings healed and in good health, you can easily communicate the same conviction to others and receive as well as minister healing with faith and boldness. **Praise be the God and father of our Lord Jesus Christ, the father of compassion and the God of all comfort who comforts us in all our troubles, so that we can comfort those in any trouble with the comfort we ourselves have received from God** (2Conrinthians 1:3&4). **For the soil which has drunk the rain that repeatedly falls upon it and produces vegetation useful to those for whose benefits it is cultivated partakes of a blessing from God** (Hebrews 6: 7 AMP.).

Once you have prayed for healing, remember that Jesus has already secured healing by His stripes (Isaiah 53:5) and that healing is God's will for you or for the one you have prayed for, then rest in the confidence that God has heard you and that His healing process has begun. Bear in mind that God is not limited with time and that sometimes He let healing come instantly and other times gradually. Usher in both instant and gradual healing and in fact anything you have prayed for according to God's will with praise and thanksgiving before you see the physical manifestation of it. Don't be discouraged and feel disappointed if the condition seems not to be improving. Be assured that God is already at work on your behalf, sending out His angels to do what is required to bring His will to pass in your situation. When God completes His work and accomplishes His will in your circumstance, nothing can change it. **In Him we were also chosen, having been predestined according to the plan of Him who works out everything in conformity with the purpose of His will** (Ephesians 1:11). **Yes from the time of the first existence of day and from this day forth, I am He; there is no one who can deliver out of my hand. I will work and who can hinder or reverse it?**

Bear in mind that as a child of God, you are saved and healed the moment you accepted Jesus Christ and received Him into your heart as your saviour. He became also your healer and by your daily surrender to the control of the Holy Spirit, He can also be the Lord of your entire life. With this mindset, you can live your Christian life from a position of power over sickness and everything the devil may throw at you. You can, through the Holy Spirit continue the works Jesus begun by confidently ministering healing to the sick. **As you go, preach this message: The kingdom of heaven is near.' Heal the sick, raise the dead, and cleanse those who have leprosy, drive out demons. Freely you have received, freely give** (Matthew 10:7-8). **When Jesus has called the Twelve together, He gave them power and authority to drive out all demons and to cure diseases and He sent them out to preach the kingdom of God and to heal the sick** (Luke 9:1&2). Jesus' disciples obeyed and carried out their assignment of miraculously healing the sick while He was still with them. When Jesus died, rose and went back to heaven, healing of the sick did not stop. His apostles continued. **There was an estate nearby that belonged to Publius, the chief officer of the island. He welcomed us to His home and for three days entertained us hospitably. His father was sick in bed, suffering from fever and dysentery. Paul went in to see him and, after prayer, placed his hands on him and healed him** (Acts 28:7&8). **As Peter travelled about the country, he went to visit the saints in Lyda. There he found a man named Aeneas, a paralytic who had been bedridden for eight years. Aeneas, Peter said to him, "Jesus Christ heals you. Get up and take care of your mat." Immediately Aeneas got up** (Acts 9:32-35).

Beatrice, a 24-year old young Christian woman from a strong Catholic background feels that healing of the sick is for the priests and some elders of the Church. After being born again few months ago, Beatrice is learning through new Christians' Bible studies that every born again Christian has been commissioned by Jesus to preach the gospel and heal the sick. **And He said to them, "Go into all the world and preach the gospel to every creature. And these signs shall follow those who believe: In my name they shall cast out demons; they will speak with new tongues; they will take up serpents ; and if they drink anything deadly, it will by no means hurt them; they will lay hands on the sick, and they will recover** (Mark 16:15,17,18). **Most assuredly I say to you, he who believes in me, the works that I do he will do also; and greater works than these he will do, because I go to My Father** (John 14:12).

On the strength of the above assurance by Jesus, Beatrice has learnt to stand her ground and lay hands by faith on herself whenever she or anyone faces a health challenge. She said, "I now strongly believe the teaching that God has forgiven all my sins and healed all my diseases as seen in psalm 103:2&3 and so whenever I am sick, I remind myself that I am already saved as well as healed."

QUESTIONS FOR REFLECTION
1. Explain in your words the statement that you give what you have in regards to receiving and ministering divine healing.
2. At what point do you think you were saved and healed?
3. What do you do before the manifestation of the healing that has been released?

NOTES

CHAPTER 12

ONLY BY FAITH

Your born again spirit is designed to commune with God who is Spirit. To be able to believe Him whom we do not see with our physical eyes, God gave each person a measure of faith with which to uniquely relate with Him person to Person. He is pleased only when you exercise your measure of faith to believe for such things as the healing of your body and for all His promises to you. **For by the grace given to me I say to every one of you: Do not think of yourself more highly than you ought, but rather think of yourself with sober judgement, in accordance with the measure of faith God has given you** (Romans 12:3). **And without faith it is impossible to please God, because anyone who comes to Him must believe that He exists and rewards those who earnestly seek Him** (Hebrews 11:6). What is faith? **Now faith is the substance of things hoped for, the evidence of things not seen** (Hebrews 11:1). **Faith comes by hearing the word of God** (Romans 10:17). This means the words that the Holy Spirit freshly speaks to your heart concerning a particular situation. That is the word that produces life. However He speaks to you, it must agree with the scripture. Always remember that. . . . **And the very words I have spoken to you are spirit and life** (John 6:63). **He has made us competent as ministers of new covenant—not of the letter but of the Spirit; for the letter kills, but the Spirit gives life** (2 Corinthians 3:6).

Only your faith in God can give you the confidence to believe that no sickness or disease is hard for Him to deliver you from, for He is the God of all flesh. **Is there anything too hard for the**

Lord . . . . ? (Genesis 18:14). **Ah Sovereign Lord, you have made the heavens and the earth by your great power and outstretched arm. Nothing is too hard for you . . . . Behold, I am the Lord, the God of all flesh: Is anything too hard for me?** (Jeremiah 32:17&27). The uncertainty in your mind as to whether God wants to heal you keeps you doubting. Fear and unbelief whisper you cannot be healed. Your analytical reason argues against the truth that Jesus took your sins and sicknesses upon Himself, considering the symptoms. Man says it is incurable, generational and impossible. God asks you—**Is there anything too hard for me?** Only faith has the right answers to this question. Faith says **. . . with man this is impossible, but with God, all things are possible** (Matthew 19:26). **. . . Everything is possible for him who believes** (Mark 9:23).

Notice the "**All**" and the **"Every"** attached to the things/thing in the above scriptures. Jesus meant what He said. He meant unlimited possibilities with God based on His unlimited power and your faith in Him and also His mercy. There is no incurable sickness as far as God is concerned. There is no hopeless situation. There is no impossible circumstance Jesus cannot victoriously handle if you put your total faith and trust in him. When this truth becomes a fresh revelation in your spirit, hope rises where naturally there seems to be no hope, your faith grows and peace fills your heart, saying to your mind, "Be still, for all is well." This faith attitude of spirit is what you need to receive your healing or any breakthrough both privately or in a corporate situation.

During one of our meetings, before I could even finish giving a word of knowledge concerning some health challenges Jesus wanted people to receive healing from, faith began to rise and a young woman interrupted me and said, "Nneka, I am healed, I am healed. While you were talking I felt a wave of warmth on my cheek and the pain stopped." We couldn't contain our joy. Another lady received an instant healing from lower abdominal pain. She said, "I have been suffering from this pain for years, but when you mentioned that Jesus wanted to give healing to someone with a lower abdominal pain, I received it and the pain instantly left." This is to the glory of Jesus, the Healer.

These testimonies are to show you that only faith and the mercy of God can release the healing blessings of God to you or to the person you are ministering to. It doesn't matter whose faith it is. God honours faith, whether yours or the faith of the sick person. Thousands of people may be in a meeting, but only few may have faith to receive from God. Crowds of people surrounded Jesus, but only one desperate woman with an issue of blood had faith to receive healing. Jesus said to her, **Daughter, your faith has healed you. Go in peace and be freed from your suffering** (Mark 5:34). Jesus said to the blind man, **Go, your faith has healed you. Immediately, he received his sight and followed Jesus along the road** (Mark 10:52).

All through His earthly ministry, Jesus responded to people's faith in Him. To the centurion who requested for healing for his servant, He said, **Go! It will be done just as you believed it would. And his servant was healed at that very hour** (Matthew 8:13). The faith of the two blind men achieved their miracle. Jesus said to them, **According to your faith will it be done unto you. And their sight was restored . . .** (Matthew 9:29).

Mrs Albert, a new Christian woman in her 50s suffered from intestinal ulcer for years until she started listening to messages on faith. As she read the New Testament, she began to understand the finished work of Jesus on her behalf. Mrs Albert said, "I am amazed at how people like me in the bible days had simple faith in Jesus and received their healing." As soon as Mrs Albert exercised her faith, she received her complete healing, though progressively. Hebrews 11 show cased men of faith. Every breakthrough, every miracle experienced and every battle won by any of them was by their own faith. Develop and exercise your own faith for only by it can you please God.

QUESTIONS FOR REFLECTION

1. Name some of the things that can easily oppose your faith for divine healing and discuss how you can overcome them.
2. What can happen within you when the truth that there is nothing impossible with God becomes a fresh revelation to you?
3. Share any healing testimony that resulted out of your personal faith to the glory of Jesus.

NOTES

CHAPTER 13

SEARCH THE SCRIPTURES

The written word of God concerning healing of any type, particularly the healing of your physical body and your mind is a revelation of His will for your wellness. When you search them out as revealed by the Holy Spirit, read, meditate and confess them over your life, your faith for healing is most likely to increase. **My son, give attention to my words; incline your ear to my saying, for they are life to those who find them, and health to all their health** (Proverbs 4:20 & 22). **Beloved, I pray that you may prosper in every way and that your (body) may keep well even as (I know) your soul keeps well and prospers** (3 John 2 AMP.). **As the rain and snow come down from heaven and do not return to it without watering the earth and making it bud and flourish so that it yields seed for the sower and bread for the eater, so is my word that goes out from my mouth: it will not return to me empty, but will accomplish what I desire and achieve the purpose for which I sent it** (Isaiah 55: 10&11).

Believe in your heart that God wants you totally healed, that He wants you to live and enjoy good health. Believe that for this reason, He gave up Jesus, His only Son so that by His stripes, you are healed. Believe it in your heart and confess daily with your mouth all the healing scriptures in this chapter and your faith for healing will increase. **For it is with your heart that you believe and are justified, and it is with your mouth that you confess and are saved** (Romans 10:10). **The good man brings good things out of the good stored**

up in his heart . . . . For out of the overflow of his heart his mouth speaks (Luke 6:45).

I like this beautiful testimony from Peter Allard's book, *NOW FAITH IS*, showing the power of believing and confessing God's ability to bring healing, despite the symptoms. Enjoy. The author reported, *"During a series of meetings some years ago, a young woman came for prayer, suffering from pyorrhea (Pyorrhea is a dental disease that affects and damages the bones around the teeth) . . . . The word leapt into my heart, "Is there anything too hard for the Lord?" We prayed then looked into her mouth. There was no apparent change . . . . But now listen to her testimony . . ."*

The lady testified, *"At first nothing happened, I went and sat back in my seat. In my mind I was saying, "Lord I know you are going to heal me. If it doesn't happen tonight, I know I will be alright in the morning. And if I'm not alright in the morning, I'll keep on believing and because I really believe, I know you will do this for me." Then it happened! It was like a shock of electricity. . . . I cried out, God is healing me!" . . . I put my tongue behind my front teeth and could feel them smoothing out. All the back teeth on the right side of my mouth had filled with silver. They shone like diamonds. By this time all the teeth on the left side had filled . . . As I write this my front teeth are still healing. The enamel is growing across and the holes are getting smaller and smaller. As I keep believing, they keep healing. I am sure He will do for you what He has done for me. The hard thing is to BELIEVE before you SEE!"*

The best thing in your walk with Jesus is to believe Him before you see the manifestation of your healing miracle and the fulfilment of His promises to you. Take time to prayerfully read the following healing scriptures, meditate on them and personalise them until they pass from your head to your heart. Keep confessing them until you see complete healing.

Exodus 15:26— **. . . . I am the Lord who heals you.** (Note that Jesus satisfied all the conditions attached to the Old Covenant. So feel free to claim this promise).

Exodus 23:25 **Worship the Lord your God, and His blessings will be on your food and water. I will take away sickness from among you.**

Psalm 91:16 **with long life will I satisfy him and show him my salvation.**

Psalm 103:3 **Praise the Lord, O my soul and forget not all His benefits-who forgives all your sins and heals all your diseases.**

Psalm 107:20 **He sent forth His word and healed them; He rescued them from the grave.**

Isaiah 53:5 **But He was pierced for our transgressions, He was crushed for our iniquities; the punishment that brought us peace was upon Him and by His wounds we are healed.**

Search the scripture for other passages on healing, meditate and believe.

QUESTIONS FOR REFLECTION

1. How do you know that God wants you and other human beings well? Discuss.
2. How can your faith for healing be increased?
3. What does it mean to live by faith in general, and especially in regards to healing?

NOTES

CHAPTER 14

COMMON-SENSE HEALTHY LIFE STYLE

C ommon-sense, according to Macquarie Dictionary is sound practical perception or understanding. In relation to this chapter, it means sound practical understanding and application of health principles as a way of life. If you are born again Christian, your body is the temple of God which requires to be kept holy. You can keep it well by understanding how it works. **Do you not know that your bodies are temples of the Holy Spirit who is in you . . . therefore honour God with your bodies** (1 Corinthians 6:19&20). **By wisdom a house is built, and through understanding it is established . . .** (Proverbs 24:3). Just as your spirit and soul prosper and are preserved by the Holy Spirit and the word of God so is your body built and preserved by what you eat and drink. I like this thought. Please note that no health expertise is claimed in this chapter. My only aim is simply to provoke some thoughts in regards to some practicable ways to live in more healthy ways. *The* provoking thoughts will focus on the following: *Food;* **drinks; physical exercise; breathing exercise; sleep/rest and emotions.**

To live in more healthy ways, we should guide our appetite toward those food that are naturally designed to nourish our bodies such as unprocessed or minimally processed grains, fruits, vegetables, nuts and all the foods that God provided for mankind. From the beginning, God gave mankind a guideline for healthful eating. **I give you every seed-bearing plant on the face of the whole earth and every tree**

that has fruit with seed in it. They will be yours for food . . . I give every green plant for food. And it was so (Genesis 1:29&30). **All the animals of the earth, all the birds of the sky . . . all the fish in the sea . . . I have given them to you for food, just as I have given you grain and vegetables** (Genesis 9:2&3). The point is that God wants you to eat foods to promote health instead of starving or eating to impair it.

Besides, you must know your body; listen to it; honour it by paying attention to what it tells you from time to time. Sometimes it tells you the foods it likes or dislikes, the amount it needs and the suitable or unsuitable time to feed it. Eat it simple, according to the season of the year; according to the kind of work you do and not according to your family tradition or culture. Never use food as comfort lest you become addicted to it and exceed your healthy weight. For more, I suggest you do some internet research on food and nutrition or talk to a local Nutritionist. Knowledge is power. Knowing your body and applying wisdom in feeding it with the kind of foods it requires to keep you going strong for the call of God in your life is a preventative measure against ill health. **A wise man is strong and is better than a strong man, and a man of knowledge increases and strengthens his power** (Proverbs 24:5 Amp.). **My people are destroyed for lack of knowledge . . .** (Hosea 4:6).

Jane, a 24 year-old dental assistant came from 4 generations of obesity and had the potential of going the way of her great grandparents, grandparents, her parents and 3 brothers and 2 sisters had she not chosen a different path. In her early teens, Jane became exposed to literature on health and nutrition. She started a campaign of healthy eating in her family but all her family members decided to stick to their family's unhealthy eating habit. Jane went it alone and today she is healthy and fit with clear skin.

What you drink also matters in keeping you healthy. Research shows that water makes up more than two thirds of the weight of the human body and without it humans would die immediately. Your body cannot function without water. Scientists assert that water lubricate your joints, regulates your body temperature; prevents or alleviates constipation; regulates your metabolism among other functions. Drinking a good amount of water each day, according to your body needs and having a daily intake of nutritious foods will keep you healthy. Besides, it is water that you need when you are thirsty for it naturally refreshes your weary and dry throat more than any other form of drink. **Daniel then said to the guard whom the chief official appointed over Daniel, Hananiah and Azariah . . . Give us nothing but vegetables to eat and water to drink. Then compare our appearance with that of the young men who eat the royal food . . . . At the end of the ten days, they looked healthier and better nourished than any of the men who ate the royal food.** (Daniel 1:11-13, 15). **He split the rocks in the wilderness and gave them water as abundant as the seas** (Psalm 78:15). Though there is no biblical command for you to drink only water, common-sense shows that pure water is safer to drink than any other drink because that was what God originally used to quench the thirst of His people as seen in the above scripture. I submit that water still remains the best thirst quencher. I am not saying that you should forbid other drinks. No. You can drink whatever you want, but always have your health at the back of your mind each time you let something go through your mouth because people say that health is wealth.

Breathing and Physical exercises are paramount to your health because they supply and generate oxygen to your body respectively. When you do more frequent abdominal deep breathing, more oxygen is released into the blood system. When you engage in physical activities, your blood circulates more and takes oxygen to various parts of your body. The oxygen in your red blood cells oxidises the food nutrients and releases energy into your body. (Thanks to my secondary school Health Science teacher). This is an elementary overview of the importance of breathing and physical exercises. There are numerous health benefits of both exercises. Do a personal search and please conduct your Doctor before embarking on any vigorous physical exercises. Though both activities are beneficial to your physical well-being and worldly gain and also demand some discipline, don't be obsessed by them or anything else and lose the eternal perspective of life. **For physical training is of some value, but godliness has value for all things, holding promise for both the present life and the life to come** (1Timothy 4:8). **Everyone who competes in the games goes into strict training. They do it to get a crown that will not last; but we do it to get a crown that will last**

forever. (1 Corinthians 9:24). In other words, let everything you do with your physical body be for the glory of God.

Sleep/physical rest and rest of mind are also important to your overall well-being because your spirit, mind and body are inter-related. One affects the other. For this reason, do what it takes to have a good rest from time to time. Allow your body to wind down and have a good restful sleep by God's grace. Ask God to bless you with sound sleep each night. He will. . . . **He grants sleep to those He loves** (Psalm 127:2NIV). **My child, don't lose sight of common sense and discernment. Hang on them, for they will refresh your soul . . . You can go to bed without fear; you will lie down and sleep soundly** (Proverbs 3:21, 22&24). Note that part of common sense is also knowing when the Lord who gives you night sleep wants you to sacrifice your night to hang out with Him or to pray for someone. In this case, be assured that as you wait in His presence, God will strengthen you in the morning and fill you with joy. **They that wait upon the Lord shall renew their strength . . .** (Isaiah 40:31). . . . **You will fill me with joy in your presence . . .** (Psalm 16:17)

QUESTIONS FOR REFLECTION

1. As a believer in Christ, why is it important to establish the well-being of your physical body?
2. What preventative measure do you need to take against ill-health?
3. Discuss the common-sense health tips and how they apply to you

NOTES

CHAPTER 15

ONE OF THE LIES OF THE DEVIL

Jesus created all things in heaven and on earth for Himself, including the angels, of which Lucifer was one. **For by Him all things were created that are in heaven and that are on earth, visible and invisible, whether thrones or dominions or principalities or powers. All things were created through Him and for Him. And He is before all things, and in Him all things consist** (Colossians 1:16&17). **In the beginning was the word and the word was with God. He was in the beginning with God. All things were made through Him, and without Him nothing was made that was made** (John 1:1-3).

Before Lucifer rebelled and was chased out of heaven and his names changed from Son of the Morning and the Anointed Cherub to devil, satan, dragon and serpent, he occupied the highest position in the Kingdom of God. **You were the anointed cherub who covers; I established you; you were on the holy mountains of God; you walked back and forth in the midst of fiery stones** (Ezekiel 28:14). **The workmanship of your timbrels and pipes were prepared for you on the day you were created** (Ezekiel 28:13a).

From being a worshiper, Lucifer became evil and hater of God and man. He is now known all over the world as the devil. One of his greatest strategies against you and the rest of mankind is deception. He deceived Eve. **You will not surely die . . . For God knows that in the day you eat of it your eyes will be opened, and you will be like God, knowing good and evil** (Genesis 3:4a &5). He can lie to you about anything, including your health and healing. **. . . the devil . . .**

He was murderer from the beginning, not holding to the truth, for there is no truth in him. When He lies, he speaks his native language, for he's a liar and father of all lies (John 8:44).

One of the Lies of the devil about sickness and disease.

Despite the truth that by the stripes of Jesus we are healed, the devil is still lying to some Christians that God allows sickness and disease to afflict their bodies to teach them some lessons and that He will surely deliver them from all of them. Such people often quote psalm 34:19 which says, **many are the afflictions of the righteous, but the Lord delivers them from them all.**

Alfonso, a 55-year old Christian man who suffers from a debilitating back pain which is compounded by a state of downcast because of an increase in pain, gathered strength on one of his bible group meetings and proudly announced, "I have faith to believe that God who allowed this affliction to come to my body, will surely heal me after He has taught me the lessons I need to learn. I believe what the bible says in Psalm 34:19 that **many are the afflictions of the righteous: but the Lord delivers them from them all.**" Alfonso got it wrong. He was deceived, maybe as a result of wrong teaching.

The word *affliction* in the context of the above Psalm in the original text is not about sickness or any physical or mental illness. It means trial, hardship, persecutions or temptation. Jesus only bore our sins and sickness and He does not want us to bear them. Full stop. On the other hand, He never promised us trouble free life because we are His. He lets us go through trials, hardships, sufferings and persecutions but promised to be with us and see us through life circumstances. So Psalm 34:19 means that these challenges may be many in the life of a believer, but the Lord will see them through. **I have told you these things, so that in me you may have peace. In this world you will have trouble. But take heart. I have overcome the world.** (John 16:33). **When you pass through the waters, I will be with you; when you pass through the rivers, they will not sweep over you. When you walk through the fire, you will not be burned; the flame will not set you ablaze** (Isaiah 43:2).

It is sad to know that some Christians like Alfonso live and die in ignorance of what is there for them in their covenant relationship with

God through Jesus. They fail to realise that under the new covenant, Jesus has already satisfied God through the cross. God is not angry with His children and will not use sickness on them as teaching aid. If you have that idea, reject it for it from the devil. Ask the Holy Spirit to give you revelations of God through the whole Bible in relation to you as the redeemed of the Lord.

In a counselling session, a 42-year old woman who presented for anger management was boasting that as a result of her husband's years of mistreatment of her, God has chastised him with a terminal lung cancer. She got the idea from Hebrews 12:6 which says, **The Lord disciplines the one He loves, and He chastens everyone He accepts as His son.**

The word *chasten* comes from a Greek word which means *instruct, train, discipline, or educate.* Though the lady agreed that she would not cause any of her children to fall sick as a way of training them, she still believed the wrong teaching that God disciplines His Children with sickness. What a lie of the devil. Don't buy into it. Use the word of God to counteract the lies of the devil in all areas of your life and live a life of victory and power on a daily basis, in Jesus' name.

QUESTIONS FOR REFLECTION

1. What was satan's initial position in heaven before his rebellion? Support answer with scriptures.
2. In the context of this chapter, what are satan's greatest strategies against you and the rest of humanity. Explain.
3. Discuss the lie satan tells about sickness as shown in this chapter. How can you handle such a lie? Share any personal experience.

NOTES

CHAPTER 16

SATAN AND DEMONS ARE UNDER YOUR AUTHORITY

I f you are a born again believer in Christ, it cannot be overemphasised that you are now the master and ruler of satan and his demons. The only place for them in your life should actually be under your feet. I like this thought that whatever they are able to get away with in the life of a Spirit filled believer or in the lives of people around them is what such believer allows in one way or another. The reason is that satan has fallen. Jesus defeated him by His death and resurrection and restored to the Church the authority Adam and Eve sold to him.

Always bear in mind that you have the power and authority from Jesus to cast out the devil and his demons. Yes they still have power but they have no authority to mess with you and the world around you because the Holy Spirit, the greater one lives in you. Demonic power is inferior to the power you possess. **But you belong to God, my children. You have already won the victory over those people, because the Spirit who lives in you is greater than the spirit who lives in the world** (1 John 4:4). Jesus said, **I saw satan fall like lightning from heaven. I have given you authority to trample on snakes and scorpions and to overcome all the power of the enemy; nothing will harm you** (Luke 10:19). **One day Jesus called together His twelve disciples and gave them power and authority to cast out all demons and heal all diseases** (Luke 9:1).

We live in a broken world where the devil easily possesses or influences people to do evil. Resist the evil one and love people by the grace of God and power of the Holy Spirit, for as a soldier of Christ, you are only called to a spiritual war against evil forces and not to attack humans. **. . . we are not fighting against flesh and blood enemies, but against evil rulers and authorities of unseen world, against mighty powers in this dark world, and against evil spirits in the heavenly places** (Ephesians 6:12). **We are humans, but we don't wage wars as humans do. We use God's mighty weapons . . . to knock down the strongholds of human reasoning and to destroy arguments. We destroy every proud obstacle that keeps people from knowing God. We capture their rebellious thoughts and teach them to obey Christ** (2 Corinthians 10:3-5).

The aim of this chapter is not to tell you what you already know, but to exhort you to always rise above whatever the devil seeks to steal, kill or destroy in your life and to remind you of where you are seated in Christ to reign in life. **And God raised us up with Christ and seated us with Him in the heavenly realms in Christ Jesus (Ephesians 2:6). And you have made them a kingdom of (royal race) and priests to our God, and they shall reign (as kings) over the earth** (Revelation 5:10 Amp.). O Hallelujah! Where you are seated spiritually is a glory expanse; a place of kingly rule where satan and his demons are under your feet as well since you are seated with Jesus; where you issue commands in the name of Jesus by the power of the Holy Spirit and all knees have no choice but to bow and submit. **What is man that you are mindful of him, the son of man that you care for him. You made him a little lower than the heavenly beings and crowned him with glory and honour. You made him ruler over the works of your hands; put everything under his feet** (Psalm 8:4-6). **Therefore God exalted Him to the highest place and gave Him the name that is above every name, that at the name of Jesus every knee should bow, in heaven and on earth and under the earth** ((Philippians 2:9&10).

Some personal proven tips that can help you stay in the place of authority and keep on reigning over the devil.

As a believer in Christ, guard your heart and mind with the assurance that all your sins are completely forgiven and God will never count it against you because of Jesus; that you have received righteousness from God. **Blessed is the man whose sin the Lord will never count against him** (Romans 4:8). **This righteousness from God comes through faith in Jesus Christ to all who believe** (Romans 3:22). Live in this mindset so that satan will not have the chance to lead you into self-righteousness, sin-consciousness, guilt and condemnation.

Another way to reign over the devil is to consciously let Jesus within you love and forgive others through your heart for without Him you can't do it. . . . . **I no longer live, but Christ lives in me** (Galatians 2:20) . . . . **apart from me you can do nothing** (John 15:5). A part from obeying Jesus, consciously chose to love and forgive and deny the devil of the chance to block the flow and personal interaction with the Holy Spirit who lives in you. Love and forgiveness do not depend on your feelings. They are just daily choices you make. Make such choices for your own health and for the sake of your relationship with God. God Himself will give you the grace if you ask Him.

Furthermore, you can live victoriously and see visions from God by guarding your heart and keeping it clean through the fire of the Holy Spirit, the blood of Jesus and the word of God. **Above all else guard your heart, for it is the wellspring of life** (Proverbs 4:23). **Blessed are the pure in heart for they shall see God** (Matthew 5:8). Form the habit of deliberately asking the Holy Spirit to purify your heart of anything that is not of Christ that can defile your heart. Sanctify every human being in your heart, knowing that they are equally loved by God and because you don't actually know their journey so far with God, just live people to God. You don't have to be friends with everyone. No. Some will like you while others will never. That's okay. Tell your brain that it's not the end of the world. God loves you already. Just let go and protect your inner world with the word of God and the blood of Jesus.

My two favourite tips which we shall look at in depth in other chapters are praise and some of the nine gifts of the Holy Spirit. They include, word of knowledge, word of wisdom, discerning of sprits and speaking in tongues. The Holy Spirit can give you a word of knowledge to know satan's schemes and a word of wisdom to know how to stay on top and not beneath and remain an overcomer. Confuse him by speaking in tongues and annoy him the more by shouting your praise to Jesus. Have fun and enjoy your life in Jesus on a daily basis in Jesus' name.

QUESTIONS FOR REFLECTION

1. Where did your authority over satan and demons come from? Support answer with scriptures.
2. What happens when you exercise your authority over the devil and his demons? What happens when you don't?
3. Discuss the author's personal tips that can help you stay in the place of authority over the devil.

NOTES

CHAPTER 17

THE POWER AND AUTHORITY IN THE WORD OF GOD

What God has spoken concerning any aspect of your life, including healing will never change. He has spoken and it is settled forever. **Forever, O Lord, your word is settled in heaven** (Psalm 119:89). **Heaven and earth will pass away, but my words will by no means pass away** (Matthew 24:3). The God who sent Jesus to bear your sin and sickness is personal. He calls Himself I and addresses you directly as you read His word. **I am the Lord who heals you** (Exodus 15:26). **Beloved, I wish above all things that you may prosper and be in health, even as your soul prospers** (3 John 2).

You experience the infallibility, the power and authority of the word of God in the area of healing and in other areas of your life when you receive it afresh from the Holy Spirit for a particular need (the rhema word); when it passes from your head down to your heart and when it mixes with faith. This is when you have believed, without any doubt that God wants you healed no matter the type of sickness; no matter the medical report. Healing takes place when it is settled both in your spirit and mind that it is Jesus Himself who heals; that deep down in His heart now, He wants all mankind to receive healing and live in good health.

This unshakeable truth gives you the confidence to receive your healing and also to release the healing power of God to the sick. He wants to satisfy you and others who believe with long life. **This is the**

confidence we have in approaching God: that if we ask anything according to His will, He hears us. And if we know that He hears us, whatever we ask, we know that we have what we ask for. (1 John 5:14&15). **With long life will I satisfy him and show him my salvation** (Psalm 91:16). **And may you live to see your children's children** (psalm 128:6). When there seems to be no hope, put your trust in Jesus Christ, and ask the Holy Spirit to breathe upon the written word for your situation and give it a life of its own. Believe in your heart and confess the word of God such as, **I shall not die, but live and declare the works of the Lord** (Psalm 118:17). **The Lord will fulfil His purpose for me** (Psalm 138: 8). Remember that one of the purposes of God for all mankind is divine health and healing as demonstrated by Jesus. . . . **how God anointed Jesus of Nazareth with the Holy Spirit and with power, who went about doing good and healing all that were oppressed by the devil, for God was with Him** (Act 10:38). **A vast crowd brought to Him people who were lame, blind, crippled, those who couldn't speak, and many others. They laid them before Jesus and He healed them all** (Matthew 15:30).

Jesus Himself is the word of God and He demonstrated His power and authority as He healed the sick. Your faith rises when you receive the word of God for a particular condition. Focus on Jesus, the word of God and the healer as you believe for healing for yourself or for those you minister to because He is the word that God sent to do His will, which included healing the sick. **For I have come down from heaven, not to do my own will, but the will of Him who sent me** (John 6:38). **He sent forth His word and healed them; He rescued them from the grave** (Psalm 107:20). Jesus is your healer. Jesus is the one who will heal those you minister to. You can guarantee the manifestation of His power and authority over sickness and diseases when you surrender to Him and let Him have His way in all aspects of your life, including receiving and ministering healing. . . . . **Do not be afraid. Stand still and you will see the deliverance the Lord will bring you today. The Egyptians you see today, you will never see again.** (Exodus 14:13). **Be still, and know that I am God; I will be exalted among the nations, I will be exalted in the earth.** (Psalm 46:10).

Anton, a 39-year-old new Christian man with a chronic migraine received an instant healing as he watched a Christian television program where a miracle healing Evangelist was inviting viewers to put their focus and trust on Jesus while He was preaching the Gospel. Anton said, *"I came from a Hindu background where they have different gods but for years none of them was able to cure me of this chronic migraine. My friend told me to watch a certain healing program on the television. I am sure if he had told me it was a Christian program, I wouldn't have bothered to tune in to that station. Well I did. I was hooked by the message and before I knew it, the intense headache left me. The preacher said, "If you are healed, jump up and shout for joy onto Jesus anywhere you are and ask Him to forgive all your sins and save you. Tell Him to come and live in you." I did and since four years I have been a committed Christian without any migraine headache again. Thank you Jesus."*

Anton's powerful message and many similar stories show that there is no time or space barrier to the healing power of Jesus. In any situation you find yourself now, I pray in Jesus' name that you find courage to lift up your head and look unto Jesus and be saved from sickness or anything that the evil one has used to oppose your life in general. Amen.

QUESTIONS FOR REFLECTION

1. When do you experience the infallibility and the authority of the word of God in your situation?
2. On whom do you focus as you meditate on the word of God or as you seek or minister healing? Explain.
3. Support with scriptures or personal testimony the statement that there is no distance with God in regards to the flow of His healing power.

NOTES

CHAPTER 18

YOUR INTERNAL DIOLOGUE

Internal dialogue means your inner conversation with yourself. What you continually say to yourself internally will always show in your body language, behaviour or speech pattern and it stems from your beliefs, especially when it comes to healing. **And behold, a woman who had suffered from a flow of blood for twelve years came up behind Him and touched the fringe of His garment. For she kept saying to herself, if I only touch His garment I shall be restored to health** (Matthew 9: 20&21). **But the Centurion replied to Him, Lord, I am not worthy or fit to have you come under my roof: but only speak the word, and my servant boy will be cured** (Matthew 8:8). The internal dialogues of the woman and the Centurion which were rooted in their belief that Jesus had the answer to their pressing needs eventually manifested in their step of faith and utterances respectively. Jesus was amazed at their faith which released His healing virtue as needed.

Whether you voice it out or not, you are always talking to yourself about different things through your thoughts and feelings and what you say from within affects your inside and outside world. That internal conversation may be thoughts, that according to Doctor's report, the sickness is incurable. It may be a conversation of feelings of anxiety, worry about your illness or that of another. It may even be fear of falling sick or being in trouble of any kind. If those inner negative dialogues continue uncounteracted by your faith, you will most likely attract the condition. **What I feared has come upon me; what I dreaded has happened to me.** (Job 3:25). **An anxious heart weighs**

a man down, but a kind word cheers him up (Proverbs 12:26). Note that if you are anxious about the sickness in your body and you have this ongoing conversation that many die from that sickness and so it is likely you will also die from it, you are already living in defeat which is against your new nature. Don't forget that in Christ you are an overcomer and more than a conqueror.

Sandy, a single 30-year-old Accountant with a prestigious Account firm and also a new Christian woman had aspirations of climbing her career ladder in her industry. However, she has this ongoing conversation within her that since most members of her father's family died suddenly of minor illnesses before the age of 40, she was most likely to die anytime of even common cold. Sandy said, *"My goal is to be an executive account manager in any firm before I depart like others."* Sandy was surprised to see that employment opportunity slipped away from her in many occasions with such statements from the companies as-"*. . . We are sorry to let you know that you are over qualified for this position."* Sometimes she got such response as, *"We think you may not stay long in the position if we hire you." ". . . Sorry this is a permanent position and we feel that it is not suitable for your current long experience."* These and other similar responses from industry executives of few other Account firms made Sandy to seek prayers and counselling. The Counsellor focused on the entire "Cycle"-defeating self-talk that produced more rejections, not only in the area of Sandy's employment but also in her relationships with the opposite sex.

The Christian Counsellor helped Sandy to understand that the industry executives were responding to her "death schedule" which she rehearsed in her head every day and not necessarily to her over qualification. During the six counselling sessions, Sandy learnt how to challenge her inner negative self-talk and to construct positive inner declarations through such word of God as—**I shall not die, but live, and declare the work of the Lord** (Psalm 118:17). **He satisfies your mouth (your necessity and desire at your personal age and situation) with good so that your youth renewed, is like the eagle's(strong, overcoming, soaring)** (Psalm 103:5 Amp.). **With long life will I satisfy and show him my salvation** (Psalm 91:16). The Counsellor worked with Sandy until she started to believe that as a Christian, all the promises in the Bile belong to her because of Jesus' finished work on the cross. As she began to search the scriptures for herself, meditating and confessing them out in regards to her situation, Sandy grew in her faith. A year later, she got a senior management position in one of the top Account firms in her state. As time went on, Sandy got more involved in her local Church, believing to end up marrying the gentle man who fell in love with her during one of their Church events.

Sandy's case is a clear example of how people can self-talk themselves into and out of things. A sick person may be having an endless conversation within why they are being prayed for. They may be saying, *"I know that by the stripes of Jesus, I am already healed and so I receive my healing in Jesus' name."* Or, the person may have concluded that their sickness is incurable and engage in such internal dialogue as, *"I can't see any way out of this one according to the medical report and more so, not many survive from this type of illness."* If you are off track, resolve to talk yourself back into what God wants for your life by meditating on, believing and confessing over your life or over the lives of others the word of God concerning your healing or other blessings of God. **So is my word that goes out from my mouth: it will not return to me empty, but will accomplish what I desire and achieve the purpose for which I sent it** (Isaiah 55:11). . . . **I am watching over my word to perform it** (Jeremiah 1:12).

QUESTIONS FOR REFLECTION

1. Explain in your own words what you understand by internal dialogue. Where does it originate from?
2. What happens when negative internal dialogue is ignored?
3. How would you challenge negative self-talk?

NOTES

Chapter 19

THE CONFESSION OF
YOUR MOUTH

The dictionary meaning of the word 'confession' is acknowledgement of something. With your mouth you acknowledge or confess what you believe or do not believe. For example, when you accepted Jesus as Lord and saviour, you not only acknowledged your sins, you acknowledged or confessed with your mouth your belief in Him and received salvation, which surely included your healing, lest you forget. **So then, brethren, consecrated and set apart for God, who share in the heavenly calling (thoughtfully and attentively) consider Jesus, the Apostle and High Priest whom we confessed (as ours when we embraced the Christian faith)** (Hebrews 3:1 AMP.). **That if you confess with your mouth, 'Jesus is Lord' and believe in your heart that God raised Him from dead, you will be saved. For it is with your heart that you believe and are justified, and it is with your mouth that you confess and are saved** (Romans 10:9&10).

What you confess is very important in regards to your healing and general well-being. This is because just as you received salvation which included the healing of your mind and body by believing in your heart and confessing Jesus with your mouth, so also can you bring or be bound by sickness in your body through unbelief and the confession of your mouth. **And He was not able to do one work of power there, except that He laid His hands on a few sickly people and cured them. And He marvelled because of their unbelief . . .**

(Mark 6:5&6). **You are snared with the words of your lips; you are caught by the speech of your mouth** (Proverbs 6:2). If you focus on and always talk about how bad your physical condition is, sickness holds you in bondage. If you keep confessing how fearful you are of your condition, fear increases its hold on you. Fear is one of satan's weapons he uses to steal, kill or destroy, not only faith in God but also human lives.

Beatrice, a 32-year-old nurse and also a Christian woman went for a minor key-hole surgery and died of fear because she kept confessing her fear of death before the procedure. She kept saying, *"I am so scared of this thing. I am afraid I will even die of the anaesthetic. Something can go wrong and I'm gone."*

A wrong confession like that of Beatrice is a defeatist approach to life situation. As a Christian, you already know that satan and his demons are forever defeated and that they are under Jesus' feet and under yours as well. When you always confess how bad things are; how the devil is having a go at you; how hopeless your situation is; how things are not changing; how things have not been working for you or your family and on and on and on, you are elevating satan and giving him the acknowledgement and supremacy he does not deserve and concretising your situation with your words. In other words, you are making your situation stay put, well rooted and immovable. As long as you cling to the confession of sickness, failure and weakness, they will remain your reality. You may listen to faith preaching and ask some men or women of faith to pray for you, but you may not see any change because your negative confessions and unbelief will hinder your faith to receive. Not only that, such negative confessions actually sap energy out of your whole being and live you dry in your inner man.

What to confess

To start with, if you are a born again Christian, believe that because of the finished work of Jesus on the cross, God the father loves you exactly the way He loves Jesus. **. . . You have loved them (even) as you have loved me** (John 17:23). **I have given them the glory and honour which you have given me** (John 17:22). Believe that God is not angry at you and will never because Jesus satisfied all

His requirements on your behalf through the cross. **To me this is like the days of Noah when I swore that the waters of Noah would never again cover the earth. So I have sworn not to be angry with you, never to rebuke you again** (Isaiah 54:9). **Having wiped out the handwriting of requirements that was against us, which was contrary to us. And He has taken it out of the way, having nailed it to the cross** (Colossians 2:14). Believe that He wants the best for you and that He wants you healed and to enjoy good health. **Dear friend, I pray that you may enjoy good health and that all may go well with you, even as your soul is getting along well** (3 John 2). **. . . . For I am the Lord who heals you** (Exodus 15:26b).

It is very important for you to grasp the meaning of the cross and let the Holy Spirit plant the truth of it deep down to your heart, lest satan uses religion to rob you of God's blessings that accompany Jesus' finished work on the cross, which include divine healing and health. Through the written word of God, you must know how God sees you in Christ, what He says about you in Christ. You must read, meditate and believe for yourself that every promise in the bible from Genesis to revelation is yours because of Jesus. Only when these truths are ingrained deep within you can you confess the word of God over situations with faith inspired by the Holy Spirit like Jesus did when tempted by satan. . . . . **It has been written . . . .** (Matthew 4:4). Note that when the Holy Spirit gives you scripture verses for your situation, He breathes on them and the letter becomes alive, quick and sharp and cuts the opposing forces in pieces. Hallelujah! For example, when the devil tempts you to focus on the symptoms of sickness, personalise the word of God that says **. . . by His stripes I am healed** (Isaiah 53:5) **. . . . He heals all my diseases** (Psalm 103). Do a research of the healing scriptures and personalise them. Confess them not only when sickness knocks on the door, but as a life style. Confess not only health scriptures, but form the habit of daily speaking the corresponding word of God and His promises over your life, your family, your children, your ministry, your career, your business and the world around you. This habit is very refreshing and a wonderful way of staying in the presence of Jesus and constructing your future to the glory of God and the perpetual defeat of the devil.

If you are ministering healing to others, still speak like Jesus and the Apostles did. Speak with confidence and faith in the power of the Holy Spirit because Jesus authorised you and every believer in Him to heal the sick. **Cure the sick, raise the dead, and cleanse the lepers . . . .** (Matthew 10:8) . . . . **they will lay their hands on the sick and they will get well** (Mark 16:18). **So He stood over her and rebuked the fever, and it left her . . . .** (Luke 4:39) . . . **In the name of Jesus Christ of Nazareth, rise up and walk . . . . And at once his feet and ankle bones become strong and steady . . . . he stood and began to walk . . . .** (Acts 3:6-8). Go ahead then, receive and minister healing by faith in the name of Jesus and the confession of the word of God through the power of the Holy Spirit. Remain healed in Jesus' name Amen.

QUESTIONS FOR REFLECTION

1. What do you understand by the confession of your mouth?
2. How significant are the words of your mouth to receiving or ministering healing to others? Discuss.
3. Why is it important to daily confess the word of God over your life and those of others?

NOTES

CHAPTER 20

A TROUBLED SOUL ALSO TROUBLES THE BODY AND SPIRIT

Y ou were created as a triune being. The real you is your human spirit. You have a soul and you live in a body. God wants you to be healed and live in divine health in these three areas of your being. **Now may the God of peace Himself sanctify you completely; and may your whole spirit, soul and body be preserved blameless at the coming of our Lord Jesus Christ** (1 Thessalonians 5:23). **Dear friend, I pray that you may enjoy good health and that all may go well with you even as your soul is getting along well** (3 John 2).

When you received Jesus as your Saviour and Lord, The Holy Spirit joined with your spirit and baptised you into Christ and into His body. To baptise means to become totally identified with something or somebody. It means to become one, to be immersed into a liquid. In other words, you became one with every believer in Christ all over the world the moment you were born again. **Or do you not know that as many of us as were baptised into Christ Jesus were baptised into His death?** (Romans 6:3). **For as many of you as were baptised into Christ have put on Christ** (Galatians 3:27). **For by one Spirit we were all baptised into one body—whether Jews or Greeks, whether slaves or free-and have all been made to drink into one Spirit** (1 Corinthians 12:13). It was your born again spirit that was saved from sin and has been sealed by the Holy Spirit for eternal salvation. Through your born again spirit, you can have a daily spirit to Spirit interaction with God the father, Jesus, the written word of God through the Holy Spirit. As a born again child of God, your spirit is holy, righteous and blameless because of the finished work of Jesus on the cross. However, when your soul is engaged in your old nature and becomes consequently troubled, doubt and unbelief and all sorts of negative emotions can enter and rob your spirit of its faith, peace and joy in Christ. To protect your spirit, your soul has to be renewed through the word of God by the Holy Spirit. **. . . throw off your old sinful nature . . . instead let the Spirit renew your thoughts and attitude** (Ephesians 4:22&23). **Like newborn babies, you must crave pure Spiritual milk so that you will grow into a full experience of salvation . . .** (1 Peter 2:2).

Your soul is the part of you that relates with your natural senses and determines how you respond to the messages from your five senses—sight, smell, taste, touch and hearing. Your soul or mind is made up of your **intellect**—that part of you which reasons, thinks or argues. You have **emotions** which are your feelings that respond to your five senses. Finally, you have a **will** which is your volition that makes your decisions or choices. Research by health professionals show that health and healing of human bodies is dependent on the well-being of the soul and that when the soul is troubled, the body is also affected.

Lena, a 28-year old married woman had embarrassing itchy rashes on and between her ten fingers for three years. No amount of medical treatment was able to cure Lena of that skin condition until the Holy Spirit brought it to her attention that she had been resentful, bitter and angry toward all her in-laws who opposed her dating her now husband. Lena repented and got healed completely. From then, she realised the danger of harboring anger and bitterness in her soul. **And don't sin by letting anger control you. Don't let the sun go down while you are still angry, for anger gives a foothold to the devil** (Ephesians 4:26&27). **The thief comes only to steal, kill and destroy, but I come that they may have life and have it in full** (John 10:10).

It is very easy for the human soul to become sick because of the past hurtful experiences which in turn adversely affect the physical body. Like the physical body, your soul needs the healing touch of the Holy Spirit. For example, you will receive healing in your soul and enjoy

God's peace by renewing your mind with the word of God. **Do not conform to the pattern of this world, but be transformed by the renewing of your mind. Then you will be able to test and approve what God's will is** (Romans 12:2). **You will guard him and keep him in perfect and constant peace whose mind (both its inclination and its character) is stayed on you, because he commits himself to you . . . .** (Isaiah 26:3).

Your **emotions** can receive the healing touch of the Holy Spirit Divine by choosing to forgive those who have hurt you. Note that this is possible only by the grace of God through the power of the Holy Spirit. Forgiveness does not come natural and so you actually need to deliberately ask Jesus to forgive through you those who have inflicted deep emotional wounds in you. **Then Peter came to Him and said, Lord, how many times may my brother sin against me and I forgive him and let go? Jesus answered him, I tell you, not up to seven times, but seventy times seven** (Matthew 18:21-22). **Bear with each other and forgive whatever grievances you may have against one another. Forgive as the Lord forgave you** (Colossians 3:13). The amount of the corrosive impact of negative emotions on your body systems cannot be over emphasised. Consequently, it calls for your immediate consideration to lay all your emotional hurts at the feet of Jesus, trusting Him to give you strength to forgive where it may be extremely hard to humanly forgive.

Furthermore, your **will** must be submitted to the rulership of the Holy Spirit for your soul to receive total healing to the glory of Jesus. This is because with your will you decide whether or not to forgive others, yourself or God, whom the devil tends to cause you to accuse for allowing your hurt. With your will, you can decide whether or not to let go or stand for your right and seek revenge; whether or not to let your canal mind run the show as it did before you became born again. When the human soul is under the government of the Holy Spirit, the individual begins to gradually die to the flesh. Don't worry. It is a gradual process. The Holy Spirit is ready to gently work with you as far as you are willing to let Him have His way over your natural self which is always at loggerheads with Him. **I say then: Walk in the Spirit, and you shall not fulfil the lust of the flesh. For the flesh lusts against the Spirit and the Spirit against the flesh; and these are contrary to one another, so that you do not do the things that**

you wish (Galatians 5:16&17). **It is the Spirit who gives life; the flesh profits nothing . . .** (John 6:63). To live in the rest that Jesus died to provide for you, consider inviting Him to all the hurtful situations in your life and lay all the hurts on Him and take His peace.

QUESTIONS FOR REFLECTION
1. Explain the truth 'you are a triune being.' Support answer with scripture
2. What constitutes your soul? Explain.
3. How can your soul become sick and consequently affect your physical body and spirit? Discuss

NOTES

CHAPTER 21

YOU CAN ONLY GIVE
WHAT YOU HAVE

Whatever you are full of will eventually flow out of you. It is just a matter of time and it does not always take long. If you have received the gospel of Jesus Christ and you believed you are saved and healed at the same time by His finished work, you will likely live out these truths as loudly as possible. For example, when the devil presents to you symptoms of the disease that Jesus already healed by His stripes, you immediately look unto the Holy Spirit who dwells in you to release His healing power so that either you or the sick person will receive the healing that is already available through the wounds of Jesus. **Then Peter said, silver and gold I do not have, but what I have I give you. In the name of Jesus Christ of Nazareth, walk. Taking him by the right hand, he helped up, and instantly the man's feet and ankles became strong. He jumped to his feet and began to walk** (Acts 3:6-8). **And Stephen, full of faith and power, did great wonders and signs among the people** (Acts 6:8).

On the contrary, if a believer in Jesus Christ does not live in the revelation that physical healing is absolutely part of the redemptive work of Jesus Christ and should be preached that way, it is most likely that such Christian will not always be in the frame of mind to receive or minister healing to the sick because they are not full of faith and expectation for the release of God's healing power. This is the kind of Christian that can easily be tempted to be sceptical about the move of the Holy Spirit in performing miraculous signs and wonders through the hands of other believers who are full of faith and the power of the Holy Ghost. This kind of Christian hides under Jesus' warning against false christs and false prophets in Matthew 24:24 and practice Phariseeism. This is a situation where people who are filled with envy, jealousy, unbelief, doubt and scepticism discredit the work of the Holy Spirit through the hands of the believers in Christ whose ministries are characterised by miraculous signs and wonders. The Pharisees accepted the Bible and would have nothing to do with the Holy Spirit that enabled Jesus in His ministry. **But the Pharisees said, "It is by the prince of demons that He drives out demons."** (Matthew 9:34). **But when the Pharisees heard this, they said, "It is only by Beelzebub, the prince of demons that this fellow drives out demons."** (Matthew 12:24). **The Jews answered Him, "Aren't we right in saying that you are a Samaritan and demon possessed?"** (John 8:48). **Many of them said, He is demon possessed and raving mad. Why listen to Him?"** (John 10: 20).

When you are filled with the Holy Spirit, with His faith, hope and love, the enduring riches as seen in 1 Corinthians 13:13, your heart is pure and you can see life from God's point of view and minister to others the daily revelations you receive from Jesus. Bear in mind that God ordained to use only the Church of Jesus Christ, that is you and other believers in Christ to divinely heal, save and disciple the world. So rise and take your given authority and begin to do the works of Jesus. **He called His twelve disciples to Him and gave them authority to drive out evil spirits and to heal every disease and sickness** (Matthew 10:1). **He said to them, "Go into all the world and preach the gospel to every creature. The one who believes and is baptised will be saved, but the one who does not believed will be condemned . . ."** (Mark 16:16 NET). **Then Jesus came up and said to them, all authority in heaven and on earth has been given to me. Therefore go and make disciples of all nations, baptising them in the name of the Father and the Son and the Holy Spirit., teaching them to obey everything I have commanded you. And remember, I am with you always, to the end of the age."** (Matthew 28:18-20).

When you live your life through a daily revelation of Jesus through the Holy Spirit and the written word of God, you are most likely to be protected from passing judgement on other believers whose theology may be a bit different from yours. The reason is that your born again spirit which is in constant interaction with the Holy Spirit will pick up His counsel to refrain from passing judgement for you don't really know what goes on behind closed doors between someone and God. Besides, when you judge, you will also be judged in like manner. **Do not judge or you too will be judged. For in the same way you judge others, you will be judged . . .** (Matthew7:1&2). **There is only one law giver and judge, He who is able to save and destroy. But who are you to judge your neighbour?** (James 4:12).

Brother Roy in his 50s was a popular healing miracle Evangelist who, perhaps forgot that the Holy Spirit is not a respecter of persons and that what He does through one, He is willing and able to do through another who is willing and available. Brother Roy fell into the temptation of discrediting what the Holy Spirit was doing through another healing Evangelist. Little did bother Roy realise that rumours were circulating in the social media that his ministry was of demonic powers, which was also a lie. I am quite convinced that the Holy Spirit, being a person will be sad to see His mighty work attributed to satan. For your safety, I encourage you to live people with God so you may not be tempted to harm God's anointed ones with your mouth. Let God be the judge and focus on your own journey. Make it a habit not to listen, read or participate in slandering the servants of God or fellow believers and their work for God because you may be grieving the Holy Spirit who works through them. I don't think that the Holy Spirit will want to work through people who talk down on His power in others. Well, that's my opinion. I live it to Him. Instead of sitting and criticising others, reach out and become hungry and thirsty for intimacy with the Holy Spirit Divine and He will reveal Himself more to you.

QUESTIONS FOR REFLECTION

1. As a believer in Christ, how would you live loudly the truth that Jesus already provided healing by His finished work when you are confronted with sickness in your body or in that of another?

2. What is the evidence that a Christian is not living in the revelation that divine healing is part of the redemptive work of Jesus?

3. a) What do you understand by Phariseeism according to the author? b) What is the danger in despising a servant of God who may be operating in the power of the Holy Spirit and how would you avoid this temptation?

NOTES

CHAPTER 22

SEE IT WITHIN, BELIEVE IT, SPEAK IT, DO IT AND HAVE IT

E very human being has both outward and inward eyes. We use our outward eyes to see and appreciate God's beautiful creation and the physical world around us. The eyes of our hearts, on the other hand are meant to be used to see the spiritual world where both the good and evil spirits operate from their respective realms.

When you became a born again Christian, the Holy Spirit joined with your spirit and from then, you began in your unique ways to have spirit to Spirit interaction with God by His Spirit. From the time of your new birth and forever, the Holy Spirit longs to communicate to your heart what He hears from the father and Jesus. **But when He, the Spirit of truth comes, He will guide you into all truth. He will not speak on His own; He will speak only what He hears, and He will tell you what is yet to come** (John 16:13). . . . **No eye has seen, no ear has heard, no mind has conceived what God has prepared for those who love Him. But God has revealed it to us by His Spirit. The Spirit searches all things, even the deep things of God** (1 Corinthians 2:9&10).

Apart from the written word of God, you can also have access to the spiritual realm through the three revelation gifts of the Holy Spirit which are **distinguishing of spirits**-which is a supernatural ability to differentiate between the Spirit of God, the human spirit and demonic spirits; **word of Knowledge**-which is a supernatural revelation by the Holy Spirit of some past or present facts about you, a person or a situation which cannot be known by human mind and **word of wisdom** which is a supernatural revelation by the Holy Spirit when the believer receives God's wisdom on what action to take in a given situation based on natural or supernatural knowledge.

As a born again Christian, your relationship with Jesus is a heart to-Heart or spirit-to Spirit relationship where the Holy Spirit can use the eyes of your heart to give you words of knowledge, words of wisdom or discerning of spirits through visions or dreams. It is very unfortunate that through formal education, many of us have learnt to live out of our heads rather than our spirit man. We tend to live more in the realm of intellectual and analytical reasoning than in the realm of visions and heart promptings.

It is beyond the scope of this book to go into details about visions or dreams, but the role of your inner eyes in your Christian faith cannot be over emphasised. Once the Holy Spirit gives you word of knowledge, word of wisdom or the ability to discern spirits in flowing pictures right within you, or even outside of you in some cases, He can help you to believe it in your heart, receive the message or promise by faith, speak it out, take action based on the revelation and consequently receive a breakthrough. It cannot be overemphasised that action must follow a revelation knowledge for change, miracle, or blessings in general to follow. **After this, the word of the Lord came to Abram in a vision: "Do not be afraid Abram, I am your shield, your very reward." . . . He took him outside and said, "Look up at the heaven and count the stars. If indeed you can count them . . . so shall your offspring be. Abram believed the Lord, and He counted it to him as righteousness** (Genesis 15:1, 5&6). . . . **I tell you the truth, the Son can do nothing by Himself; He can do only what He sees His Father doing because whatever the Father does the Son also does** (John 5:19&20). **But don't just listen to God's word. You must do what it says. Otherwise, you are only fooling yourselves** (James 1:22). . . . **Faith without works is dead** (James 2:17).

Be assured that when you offer your imagination where your inner eyes are located to the Holy Spirit and ask Him to anoint and use to the glory of Jesus, He can cause you to have actual spiritual encounters with the Father, Jesus and angels in form of visions or dreams in your mind. **In the first year of Belshazzar, king of Babylon, Daniel had a dream and visions passed through his mind as he was lying on his bed** (Daniel 7:1). . . . . **an angel of the Lord appeared to Him in a dream and said, "Joseph son of David, do not be afraid to take Mary home as your wife because what is conceived in her is from the Holy Spirit** (Matthew 1:20). God has already made it possible by the Holy Spirit for you to see visions and dream revelatory dreams in these last days. He is willing to open your spiritual eyes if you can ask in faith. **In the last days, I will pour out my Spirit upon all people. Your sons and daughters will prophesy. Your young men will see visions, and your old men will dream dreams** (Acts 2:17). **I pray also that the eyes of your heart may be enlightened in order that you may know the hope to which he has called you . . .** (Ephesians 1:18).

When the Holy Spirit gives you word of knowledge and word of wisdom in flowing pictures as you minister healing to the sick, be courageous to flow with the Holy Spirit and do what you see Jesus doing. Brother Evans said, *"When I have word of knowledge or word of wisdom in flowing pictures concerning a sick person I minister to and say or do exactly what I see Jesus doing, I easily get discouraged when I don't see instant result."* Brother Evans, remember that we do not walk by sight but by faith. Always remember that you are just a yielded instrument in the hand of the Holy Spirit. He knows how and when to bring complete healing as soon as He releases His healing power through you. Healing may take place immediately or progressively. Yours is just to obey and believe.

QUESTIONS FOR REFLECTION
1. Apart from the written word of God, how else, as a believer in Christ can you receive revelation knowledge? Discuss.
2. How can the revelation knowledge you receive produce the required result ?
3. How is it possible for you to have real spiritual encounters in your mind with the Father, the Son and the angels? Support answer with scriptures.

NOTES

CHAPTER 23

BELIEVE AND REMAIN HEALED

Divine healing is the will of God expressed in His written word. **Beloved, I wish above all things that you may prosper and be in health, even as your soul prospers** (3 John 2). **For I am the Lord who heals you** (Exodus 15:26b). If you believe that God passionately wants the sick to recover, you will put your faith in the word of God and ignore the evidence of your sight, hearing and feeling in regards to the physical conditions of the sick person you are ministering to or in your own physical condition if you are the one concerned. No one will suggest that believing for healing is that naturally easy, especially when the situation is critical. Sometimes you may struggle to believe and there are other times when faith suddenly wells up from your inner recesses so much that you cannot help but believe strongly that your breakthrough has come. This extraordinary belief is the manifestation of the **gift of faith** by the Holy Spirit, which is a special ability to believe, even when a situation looks impossible. This gift is available within you the moment you receive the baptism in the Holy Spirit. It is a dynamite power within you which the Holy Spirit waits to release when it is most needed. **Not by strength and not by power, but by my Spirit, says the Lord who rules over all** (Zechariah 4:6). **. . . The Holy Spirit will come upon you and the power of the Most High will overshadow you. So, the holy one to be born will be called the Son of God. Even Elizabeth your relative is going to have a child in her old age, and she who was said to be barren is in her sixth month for nothing is impossible with God** (Luke 1: 35-37).

Apart from the critical situation where the gift of faith is required, you can live in the truth that you are already healed despite the symptoms, just as you live in the truth that you are already saved despite your short comings. **But He was wounded for our transgressions, He was bruised for our guilt and iniquities; the chastisement (needful to obtain) peace and well-being for us was upon Him, and with His stripes (that wounded) Him we are healed and made whole** (Isaiah 53:5). **Forget not all His benefits: who forgives all your iniquities; who heals all your diseases** (Psalm 103:2&3). You can believe and remain in the mental attitude of having been healed when you possess God's type of faith which is based on His word and His character with the conviction that it is impossible for Him to lie. Be mindful that you will eventually have what you believe (Good or bad). **So God has given both His promise and His oath. These two things are unchangeable because it is impossible for God to lie** (Hebrews 6:18 NLT). **And Jesus said to the Centurion, "Go; it shall be done for you as you have believed." And the servant was healed that very moment** (Matthew 8:11). **What I feared has come upon me; what I dreaded has happened to me**.

Patrick, a 45-year-old man suffered from a spinal condition for four years. He was in the habit of going from one healing crusade to another as far as a "mighty miracle evangelist" would be on the stage. Patrick would feel ecstatic as soon as he felt better and would become miserable again the next day when the symptoms showed up. He said to his home Bible study leader, *"I always feel wonderfully healed at these anointed crusades and suddenly the symptoms returned almost the following day and I would be in pain until another miracle crusade. What do you think is the problem?"* Patrick's Bible study leader replied, *"Patrick, I am happy to guide you through the scriptures concerning healing and well-being so you can develop and live by your own faith rather than on someone else's.*

After that conversation with him, Patrick's Bible study leader took him through various healing scriptures. It was not easy in the beginning because Patrick came from generations of Roman Catholic background where the Bible was originally available only to the Priests. Consequently, he grew up not knowing how to get into the scriptures through the shining light of the Holy Spirit to develop his own measure of faith even when he became born again. Not only did his faith for healing grow as time went on by meditating on the healing scriptures as revealed by the Spirit, within few months, Patrick formed the habit of daily Bible reading using a daily Bible guide given to him by his leader. It may interest you to know that Patrick received his complete healing by his own faith based on the truth that healing came together with his salvation. With that mindset, Patrick became passionate about praying for the sick with many results.

When you know who you are in Christ, your right and privileges in Him and the authority you have over the devil and his lies, you will stand your ground against his strategies to rub you of your healing. Sometimes the devil's strategy may not be unbelief or lack of personal faith as in the case of Patrick. Satan often uses the door of sin in general to get access not only to the human soul but the physical body. Life of sin may include bitterness and anger, inability to forgive others, oneself or to quit murmuring against God. All these can lead to serious mental and physical health issues that often block one from receiving healing. **Afterward, when Jesus found him in the temple, He said to him, see you are well. Stop sinning or something worse may happen to you** (John 5:14). **Just then some people brought to Him a paralytic lying on a stretcher. When Jesus saw their faith, He said to the paralytic, "Have courage son. Your sins are forgiven."** Note that as a born again Christian, all your sins are already forgiven. However, there are still adverse effects of reckless living on your mind and physical body. You can be protected daily by submitting your whole life to the control of the Holy Spirit, asking Him to purify you with His fire and the word of God. Allow the blood of Jesus to purify you of any negative emotions that can easily cause sickness in your body. Ask the Holy Spirit to give you the strength to forgive others and to forgive yourself.

QUESTIONS FOR REFLECTION
1. What kind of faith can you suddenly receive for healing when the situation looks impossible?
2. How can you develop the mental attitude that you are already healed despite the symptoms?
3. a) What other door can satan use to get sickness into your soul or body.
   b) How can you resist the devil in the context of this chapter?

NOTES

CHAPTER 24

RIGHT STANDING WITH GOD

One of the greatest weapons the devil uses to prevent some believers in Christ from receiving divine healing or creative miracles for that matter is a doubt in their minds as to whether or not they are still in right standing with God, especial during sickness, or when they miss the mark. Each time such Christians fall sick, they are tempted to think they are out of relationship with God or that they must have done something wrong that made God to allow the sickness to attack their bodies. What a lie from the pit of hell! Don't be like this type of Christian, my friend. As long as this doubt exists in a believer's mind, perfect confidence in the finished work of Jesus cannot exist; and until confidence is exercised, without doubt or double mind, the person may never feel loved, forgiven and in right standing with God while they are sick.

If you are a child of God, resolve to live, reign in life and over sickness through the grace of God without trying to establish your own righteousness. This is because your right standing with God does not depend on the things you do right. It depends totally on Jesus Christ's sacrifice of Himself on the cross by which you received righteousness or a right standing with God as a gift. **For ignoring the righteousness that comes from God, and seeking instead to establish their own righteousness, they did not submit to God's righteousness** (Romans 10:3) **For if by the transgression of the one man, death reigned through the one, how much more will those who receive the abundance of grace and of the gift of righteousness reign in life through the one, Jesus Christ** (Romans 5:17).

Jerry said, "I know it in my head that Jesus died and took away my sins and made me right with God, but sometimes, I feel so unholy and unworthy before God, especially when I am sick or each time I face one disappointment after another." Jerry continued, "At such difficult times, I feel very far from God and wonder why I have to suffer the curse of disappointments in some areas of my life even after praying." I believe Jerry spoke the mind of many Christians who for one reason or the other have not fully grasp the truth of their oneness with Christ, that God loves them exactly the same way He loves Jesus and that they were crucified, buried and raised with Christ. These Christians also need to understand that they are expected to reign in life as kings where they do not have to cower under pressure. **I in them and you in me— that they may be completely one, so that the world will know that you sent me, and you have loved them just as you have loved me** (John 17:23). **I have been crucified with Christ, and it is no longer I who live, but Christ in me. So the life I now live in the body, I live because of the faithfulness of the Son of God, who loved me and gave Himself for me** (Galatians 2:20). **Therefore we have been buried with Him through baptism into death, in order that just as Christ was raised from death through the glory of the father, so we too may live a new life** (Romans 6:4). **For He raised us from the dead along with Christ and seated us with Him in the heavenly realms because we are united with Christ Jesus** (Ephesians 2:6).

For somebody like Jerry to move from head to heart in their Christian journey, they need to surrender their entire brain and reasoning capacity to the Holy Spirit and allow Him to take the truth about their healing, their salvation, who they are in Christ and their right standing with God from their minds to their hearts. Only then can they be free to live and enjoy their Christian life. **But when He, the Spirit of truth comes, He will guide you into all truth. He will not speak on His own; He will speak only what he hears, and He will tell you what is yet to come** (John 16:13). **If you hold to my teaching, you are really my disciples. Then you will know the truth, and the truth will set you free** (John 8:31&32). Only when you know the truth that you are forever forgiven, healed by the stripes of Jesus, loved and in right standing with God through Jesus, can you have the boldness to stand your ground and rebuke satan when he attempts to cause you to feel out of relationship with God.

Always remember that the devil thrives in the ignorance or spiritual laziness of some believers in Christ who do not know what the Bible says about them and about him, the devil. Satan knows he is already defeated. He knows that even a newly born again Christian has absolute power and authority over him. He knows that divine healing is part of Jesus' redemptive work for you. He knows that as soon as the truths in the Bible sink deep within your heart through fresh revelation by the Holy Spirit, he is in trouble. The simple reason is because he can't get you to doubt your stand with God, your divine healing and his shameful defeat by Jesus. Consequently, he does everything to prevent you from meditating on the word of God. Shun his bluff and declare boldly to satan who you are and what you have in Christ Jesus, for you are the redeemed of the Lord.

For the sake of your well-being and for the glory of the father, Jesus paid the price with His precious blood and destroyed satan and his works and made you right with God. **For this purpose the Son of God was manifested, that He might destroy the works of the devil** (1 John 3:8). **Having spoiled principalities and powers, He made a show of them openly, triumphing over them in it** (Colossians 2:5).

QUESTIONS FOR REFLECTION
1. What would you tell a believer in Christ, who because they are sick, doubts whether or not they are in right standing with God?
2. In your own words, describe what life would be like for a born again Christian who lives in self-righteousness.
3. How would you minister grace to such a believer?

NOTES

CHAPTER 25

EARTHEN VESSEL

W e have already established in a previous chapter that you are a triune being. You are a spirit, you have a soul and you live in a body. Your body is an earthen vessel designed not only to house your spirit and soul, but to house the Holy Spirit from where He seeks to display His power. For this reason, God desires that this earthen vessel be dedicated for His service. **But we have this treasure in earthen vessels, which the excellency of the power may be of God and not of us** (2 Corinthians 4: 7KJV). **I appeal to you therefore, brothers, by the mercies of God, to present your bodies as a living sacrifice, holy and acceptable to God, which is you spiritual worship** (Romans 12:1).

When you sacrifice your body to God, it ceases to be yours. It then belongs to God. It is up to Him to do whatever He pleases with it. Jesus is a perfect example of a total sacrifice to His father. **So when He came into the world, He said, sacrifice and offering you did not desire, but a body you prepared for me. Whole burnt offering and sin-offerings you took no delight in. Then I said, here I am: I have come-it is written of me in the scroll of the book-to do your will, O God** (Hebrews 10:5-7). **Therefore, be imitators of God as dearly loved children and live in love, just as Christ also loved and gave himself for us, a sacrificial and fragrant offering to God** (Ephesians 5:1&2). Do not be afraid to give your mortal body to God to use as He wills and be assured that He will preserve it and quickens or restores it to health when sickness attacks it. **Moreover, if the Spirit of the one who raised Jesus from the dead lives in you, the one who**

raised Christ from the dead will also make your mortal body alive through His Spirit who lives in you (Romans 8:11). **. . . how God anointed Jesus of Nazareth with the Holy Spirit and with power, who went about doing good and healing all who were oppressed by the devil, for God was with Him** (Acts 10:38). Believe that as you surrender your whole body as an instrument for righteousness, you will, by the grace of God enjoy divine healing and good health as you serve Him with your body. Have a positive mental attitude that you will always be protected from seasonal sicknesses, such as common cold or flu. Expect the Holy Spirit to always quicken your mortal body and protect you from old age sicknesses.

There is power in expectation. Many people fall sick during winter period because they expect to be sick during cold seasons. Others expect certain illnesses as they advance in age and they have them. Some parents expect certain sicknesses to attack their infants and that often becomes their reality. Some parents of teenagers expect their young people to be depressed and suffer mood swing and they often watch their youth go down the pit of depression. Now that you know how powerful expectation is, you can make a mental shift and expect to live abundant life all through your life time, believe it and speak, take necessary actions and it shall be so for you. In the name of Jesus and through the power of the Holy Ghost, resist the spirit of fear that causes you to expect ill health and it will flee. **The thief comes only to steal and kill and destroy; I have come that they may have life, and may have it abundantly** (John 10:10). **I tell you the truth, if someone says to this mountain, be lifted up and thrown into the sea, and does not doubt in his heart, but believes that what he says will happen, it will be done for him** (Mark 11:23). The problem is not always in saying but in believing without doubt.

Christopher is a 65-year-old Christian missionary to India who suffered physical ill health while in the mission field. He reluctantly returned to his country of origin to receive some treatment with the hope to go back to India in the shortest possible time. Christopher's inability to return to the mission field due to prolonged ill health caused him some heart ache that developed into severe depression. Consequently, his speeches became negative. He said to his 25-year-old nephew "I knew it long time ago that at this age I would not be able to do any more mission trips and work as I did when I was young." He continued, "I expected that runny stomach the moment I ate certain food in India. I can as well go and be with the Lord, after all my old man died at 60." Christopher went on and on until his nephew started reminding him of how powerfully God used him in the past and how God also healed him in the past. Christopher's nephew, a dynamic youth leader was able to point him back to Jesus through the word of God he shared with him day and night. One of those days, Christopher received a total healing of his body and mind after his nephew laid hands on him and took authority over the evil one. Christopher resolved to expect long life and good health based on God's promises to His servants. He eventually returned to the mission field where he continued to do exploit for God.

Like Christopher, resolve to let the word of God lift you up on your feet when you are down, weak or doubtful. Like Christopher's nephew, build yourself up with the word of God and be strong on the inside for the sake of the weak in faith, the sick and the oppressed and be ready to step in and bring hope, encouragement and healing as the Lord gives you the opportunity.

QUESTIONS FOR REFLECTION

1. How important is your physical body and why do you think God requires you to offer it as a living sacrifice?
2. When you freely offer your body to God, what do you expect in return from Him? Explain.
3. "There is power in expectation." Elaborate in the context of this chapter.

NOTES

CHAPTER 26

YOUR PRAISE OF HIM AND HIS GLORY

To praise means to commend, to applaud, or to exalt. God is the only person that has the power and authority to say—"Look at me and all I have done and praise me. Praise me, praise me all my creations in heaven, earth and the seas." Why? The reason is because He is God. **Let the heavens and the earth praise Him, along with the seas and everything that swims in them** (Psalm 69:34) . . . . **Blessed is He who comes, the king in God's name! All's well in heaven! Glory in the high places! Some Pharisees from the crowd told Him, "Teacher, get your disciples under control!" But He said, "If they kept quiet, the stones would do it for them, shouting praise** (Luke 19:38-40 MSG).

You are now the royal priest of God anointed to praise Him if you are a child of God. In your praise of Him, you draw close to God and He fills your atmosphere with His glory or His mighty presence. **But you are a chosen people, a royal priesthood, a holy nation, God's special possession, that you may declare the praises of Him who called you out of darkness into His wonderful light** (1 Peter 2:9). **By Him therefore let us offer the sacrifice of praise to God continually, that is the fruit of our lips, giving thanks to God** (Hebrews 13:15). **But you are holy, enthroned in the praises of Israel** (Psalm 22:3 NLT). When you invite and allow the Holy Spirit to commend, applaud and magnify the father and Jesus through your lips and all that is within you, He takes over and focuses your attention on God, His majesty, His love, His mercy, His faithfulness and all that He is and does. Through the Holy Spirit, you can be lost in the presence of the Almighty God, rejoicing despite sickness or the challenges of life. When you try to praise God on your own especially in difficult times like in sickness, the flesh will not let you because of the physical or emotional pain you may be experiencing. However, when you surrender to the Holy Spirit, He takes over, renews your inward man and praises God though the outward man may be languishing in pain. It is only by the Holy Spirit can a person magnify Jesus or bear praise as the fruit of their lips in sickness or in hardship. **Therefore we do not lose heart. Even though our outward man is perishing, yet the inward man is being renewed day by day** (2 Corinthians 4:16). **Not by might nor by power, but by my Spirit, says the Lord Almighty** (Zechariah 4:6). **I am the vine; you are the branches. If you remain in me and I in you, you will bear much fruit; apart from me you can do nothing** (Matthew 15:5).

The secret of Christian living lies in intimacy with the Holy Spirit as a person. In your daily friendship with Him, you can ask Him to reveal Himself to you just as He reveals Jesus to you. As your relationship with the Holy Spirit deepens, you can begin to know His heart, His will, His emotions and in fact His ways as a person distinct from God the Father and God the Son. He will be teaching, guiding and instructing you besides other things He does. The more you listen and follow Him, the sweeter your fellowship with Him will become because He finds you capable of handling what He can offer. He also delights to share in your highs and lows. With this type of intimacy, it can become natural for you to totally surrender to the Holy Spirit Divine to do things through you. Cultivate this lifestyle and you will begin to enjoy the peace of Jesus Christ which passes all human understanding, even in sickness or in the middle of difficult situations and circumstances.

When the Holy Spirit takes over, every part of you wants to praise and worship God. You rejoice the heart of God as you praise Him for He is looking for those that can worship Him this way. There is no special qualification or instrument required by God from His children before they could praise and worship Him. All that God wants is your spirit's interacting with Him in adoration through the Holy Spirit. **Yet a time is coming and has now come when the true worshippers will worship the father in Spirit and in truth, for they are the**

kind of worshippers the father seeks (John 4:23). **Therefore, since we are receiving a kingdom that cannot be shaken, let us be thankful, and so worship God acceptably with reverence and awe** (Hebrews 12:28).

When you praise and worship God the father and God the Son, Jesus Christ by the power of the Holy Spirit despite the sickness in your body, He lifts your eyes away from the symptoms to the greatness of Jesus, causing satan and his demons to flee with their lies and suggestions about your physical or emotional conditions. Note that satan and demons are frustrated and tormented by your praise and worship of God because God dwells in the praise of His people. The devil and his demons have no choice but to flee the presence of Jesus because they are scared of being thrown into their everlasting place of torment any time. **They cried out, "Son of God, leave us alone! Have you come here to torment us before the time?"** (Matthew 8:29) **The devil who fooled them, was thrown into the lake of burning sulphur. That is where the beast and the false prophet had been thrown. They will all suffer day and night forever and ever** (Revelation 20:10).

Resolve to invite the Holy Spirit to help you to praise, worship and give thanks to God in every situation, in sickness, in health, in good and in not so good time for giving thanks like this is the will of God. When you do that, God works on your behalf and fights the devil on your behalf. **In everything give thanks; for this is the will of God in Christ Jesus concerning you** (1 Thessalonians 5:18). **And at midnight, Paul and Silas prayed and sang praises unto God and the prisoners heard them. And suddenly there was a great earthquake, so that the foundations of the prison were shaken and immediately all the prison doors were opened and everyone's bands were loosed** (Acts 16: 25&26).

Bridget, a 45-year-old pastor was diagnosed with breast cancer, but despite the report, she chose the report of the word of God that says she has been healed by the stripes of Jesus. Bridget co-operated with the Holy Spirit and praised Jesus for healing her. She saturated her mind and environment with the word of God for healing and the praise of Jesus as she received medical attention. To God be all the glory and thanks giving because this mighty woman of God received her complete healing from breast cancer and remains healed and in good health.

QUESTIONS FOR REFLECTION

1. Why is it that only God can ask for His own praise and worship?
2. Why is it important to depend on the Holy Spirit to praise and worship God?
3. What happens generally, especially in sickness when the Holy Spirit helps you to praise and worship God?

NOTES

CHAPTER 27

PREPARING THE WAY FOR THE GLORY OF THE LORD

The glory of the Lord is the tangible or weight of His presence which you can bear witness to—His love, His intervention, His provision, His character, His nature, His perfection, His might. In fact, God's glory is the display of Himself in any way He chooses so people can recognise and stand in awe of Him.

You can prepare the way for the glory of the Lord in your personal life by submitting your entire life to the Holy Spirit to work on you on a daily basis so you can grow from glory to glory. **Therefore I urge you, brothers and sisters, in view of God's mercy, to offer your bodies as a living sacrifice, holy and pleasing to God—this is your true and proper sacrifice** (Romans 12:1 NIV). **Make a straight highway through the wasteland for our God. Fill in the valleys, and level the mountains and hills. Straighten the curves, and smooth out the rough places. Then the glory of the Lord will be revealed, and all people will see it together. The Lord has spoken** (Isaiah 40:3-5). **So all of us who have had that veil removed can see and reflect the glory of the Lord. And the Lord who is Spirit—makes us more and more like Him as we are changed into His glorious image** (2 Corinthians 3:16).

When you allow the Holy Spirit to help you grow from glory to glory, you will eventually come to a stage where you begin to share the heart cry of God for the lost humanity, which is to save everyone from the power of sin. **This is good and pleases God our Saviour**

who wants everyone to be saved and to understand the truth (1 Timothy 2:3&4) **The Lord is not slow in keeping His promise, as some understand slowness. Instead He is patient with you, not wanting anyone to perish, but everyone to come to repentance** (2 Peter 3:9 NIV). People at this stage agree with Jesus that it is time for the harvest of the lost humanity and they are willing to be sent to the field. **You may know the saying, 'Four months between planting and harvest.' But I say, wake up and look around. The fields are already ripe for harvest** (John 4:35) . . . . **The harvest is great, but the workers are few. So pray to the Lord who is charge of the harvest; ask Him to send more workers into the fields** (Mathew 9:37&38).

Note that as far as Jesus is concerned, every believer in Him has been commissioned to go to the harvest fields, beginning from your immediate world to the nations of the world and demonstrate His power and glory and bring people back to God. **Peace be with you. As the father sent me, I am sending you** (John 20:21). **Therefore go and make disciples of all the nations, baptizing them in the name of the Father and the Son and the Holy Spirit** (Matthew 28:19) **For as the waters fill the sea, the earth will be filled with the awareness of the glory of the Lord** (Habakkuk 2:14).

To prepare the way for the knowledge of glory God to fill the earth, you need to identify your sphere of influence and take ownership of it first by prayer and fasting as led by the Holy Spirit. I believe that figuratively speaking, your sphere of influence is your 'land' on which God wants to manifest His glory. In other words, He wants everyone in that sphere to be aware of His glory. This means the invasion of His reality in people's individual lives through the Holy Spirit. In his book, THE SECRET PLACE, William J. Dupley listed what Loren Cunningham described as society's spheres of influence which are also known as seven mountains. They are:

1. Religion
2. Family
3. Education
4. Government
5. Media and Communication
6. Arts and Entertainment
7. Business

You are definitely called to any of or some of these spheres. Know that they are your 'lands.' Ask the Holy Spirit to give you words of knowledge to know the past and present situation of things. Ask for the gift of discerning of spirits so you can know what spirits rule in that territory or territories. Ask the Holy Spirit to give you word of wisdom to know how to pray, what action to take, when and how.

When you receive the revelation knowledge about your 'land', then pray with compassion and love for the lost, never judging or condemning them, but asking God to forgive and have mercy on the sinner as you pray. This is because Jesus did not come to judge the world but to save it (John 3:17). Fast when you are led by the Holy Spirit. Exercise your spiritual authority by binding and casting out the ruler demons in those territories. Be militant and violently take the 'land' from the devil and loose the manifestation of the glory of God in that or those areas. Go about your normal duties in the confidence that the Holy Spirit is already touching people's hearts through your prayers before you arrive at the harvest fields. **If my people, who are called by my name, will humble themselves and pray and seek my face and turn from their wicked ways, then I will hear from heaven, and I will forgive their sin and will heal their land** (2 Corinthians 7:14). **I will go before you and level the mountains; I will break down gates of bronze and cut through bars of iron** (Isaiah 45:2).

QUESTIONS FOR REFLECTION

1. What in your own words is the glory of the Lord?
2. How can you prepare for the daily manifestation of the glory of the Lord in your life?
3. a) List the seven society's spheres of influence according to Loren Conningham.

   b) How can you prepare for the knowledge of the glory of the Lord in your own sphere or spheres of influence?

NOTES

CHAPTER 28

WORKING LIKE JESUS

With the conviction that we have been permitted by Jesus as believes in Him to do the works He did and to do even more, it goes without saying that we should seek to work like Him. Every work that Jesus did during His earthly ministering was founded on the love and compassion of God for humanity and obedience to the will of His father. **Moved with compassion, Jesus reached out and touched him. "I am willing," he said. "Be healed!" Instantly the leprosy disappeared, and the man was healed** (Mark 1:41&42). **When the Lord saw her, His heart overflowed with compassion. "Don't cry!" He said. Then he walked over to the coffin and touched it . . . "Young man," He said, "I tell you, get up." Then the dead boy sat up and began to walk! And Jesus gave him back to his mother** (Luke 7:13-15).

Being moved by and engaged in alleviating human suffering, Jesus was demonstrating the will of His father who sent Him. **Then Jesus explained: "My nourishment comes from doing the will of God who sent me, from finishing His work** (John 4:34). **Father, if you are willing please take this cup of suffering away from me. Yet I want your will to be done, not mine** (John 22:42). Remember that it is the will of God to heal the sick, no matter who. Don't forget that. This calls for you to minister with confidence and with compassion, knowing that you are doing the will of God. James said, "I don't always feel compassionate towards people and so, when I see sick or poor people, I am not usually moved like Jesus. Is anything wrong with me?" James, remember that there is no more condemnation for those in Christ

Jesus, as Paul said in Romans 1:8. I will assure you that Jesus does not condemn you, neither should you condemn yourself. I believe that as you grow in Christ, you will also grow in the love of God which the Holy Spirit has poured in your heart. One day at a time until His compassion flows in great measure with His love. You can even ask the Holy Spirit to begin to quicken this process and empower you to go out with compassion and serve humanity as Jesus did, for the harvest is great.

Though Jesus was fully God, He gave up His glory and privileges as God and took the human form. He depended totally on His father through the Holy Spirit in His earthly ministry. **Who being in every nature God, did not consider equality with God something to be used to His own advantage; rather, He made himself nothing by taking the very nature of a servant, being made in human likeness** (Philippians 2:6&7). **For in Christ lives all the fullness of God in human body** (Colossians 2:9). **When all the people were being baptised, Jesus was baptised too. And as He was praying, heaven was opened and the Holy Spirit descended on Him in bodily form like a dove . . . .** (Luke 3:21&22). **Jesus returned to Galilee in the power of the Spirit . . .** (Luke 4:14). **One day Jesus was teaching, and the Pharisees and teachers of the law were sitting there . . . And the power of the Lord was with Jesus to heal the sick** (Luke 5:17).

Always remember that as a Spirit baptised believer in Christ, ministering to the sick or doing other works that Jesus did, like preaching and teaching must always be by the power of the Holy Spirit. That is the only way you are meant to be an effective witness of Jesus Christ. This reminder cannot be overemphasised because Christian ministry outside the Holy Spirit is strenuous and fruitless . . . **Not by might, nor by power, but by my Spirit, says the Lord** (Zechariah 4:6). **But you shall receive power when the Holy Spirit comes on you; and you will be my witnesses in Jerusalem, and in all Judea, and Samaria, and to the ends of the earth** (Acts 1:8).

Clifford, a 35-year-old Christian man is concerned that sometimes He is confused as to when the Holy Spirit is leading and when it is him taking the decision to pray for the sick, give a word of encouragement or operate in some gifts of the Holy Spirit.

My response to Clifford is to keep on cultivating an intimate relationship with the Holy Spirit because He will be dealing with you in a unique way like He does with every person on earth. By daily acknowledging and honouring Him as God, letting Him know of your daily dependence on Him and actually talking to Him like you do to the father and Jesus, you begin to develop a deeper intimacy with this marvellous Holy Spirit Divine so much so that you can rarely mistake His voice or His movement in your heart. Consequently, you can begin to work as He directs you. Jesus depended on the Holy Spirit to see what the father was doing or saying so that He could do the same. **I tell you the truth the Son can do nothing by Himself. He does only what He sees the Father doing. Whatever the Father does, the Son also does** (John 5:19). **My message is not my own; it comes from God who sent me** (John 7:16).

QUESTIONS FOR REFLECTION
1. What was the foundation of Jesus' earthly ministry?
2. What would you do to become familiar with the way the Holy Spirit uniquely communicates with you?
3. In regards to healing ministry, how important is the leading of the Holy Spirit to you? Explain.

NOTES

CHAPTER 29

JESUS IS WILLING TO USE YOU IF YOU ARE

Jesus sought to duplicate Himself through His twelve apostles and other disciples, and He did. He also wanted others who were not yet involved in extending the Kingdom of God to be recruited into the harvest field. Jesus was all out to bring as many people as possible to the kingdom of God. **Jesus called His twelve disciples together and gave them authority to cast out evil spirits and to heal every kind of disease and illness** (Matthew 10:1). . . . **I have been given all authority in heaven and earth. Therefore, go and make disciples of all the nations, baptising them in the name of the Father and the Son and the Holy Spirit** (Matthew 28:18&19). **I have other sheep too that are not in this sheep fold. I must bring them also. They will listen to my voice, and there will be one flock with one shepherd** (John 10:16). **The Lord appointed seventy-two others and sent them two by two . . . He told them, the harvest is plentiful, but the workers are few. Ask the Lord of the harvest, to send out workers into His harvest field** (Luke 10: 1&2).

Jesus is willing to recruit and use you to preach the gospel, heal the sick and bring many to the kingdom of God if you are willing and available. The moment you became born again, you received the command to preach the Good News of the kingdom of God and minister healing to the sick no matter your occupation. So it's not a matter of God's willingness to use you but your willingness to be used. **Go into all the world and preach the gospel to all creation . . .**

And these signs will follow those who believe: In my name they will cast out demons; they will speak with new tongues; they will take up serpents; and if they drink anything deadly, it will by no means hurt them; they will lay hands on the sick, and they will recover (Mark 16:15, 17&18). **And this gospel of the kingdom will be preached in all the world as a witness to all the nations and then the end will come** (Matthew 24:14).

Jesus is not only willing to use you to preach the gospel and heal the sick, He is also willing to use you to serve Him by serving humanity in the areas He has called and gifted you if you are willing. **For we are God's handiwork, created in Christ Jesus to do good works, which God prepared in advance for us to do** (Ephesians 2:10). **Whatever you do, work at it with all your heart, as working for the Lord . . . It is the Lord you are serving** (Colossians 3:23&25).

Clifford was a 24-year-old enthusiastic new Christian who read his Bible and some Christian literature alongside some self-help materials that emphasised that everyone should strive to get the most out of life. Consequently, the young Clifford would do whatever it took to attend this service and that service; this conference and that conference; receiving and receiving the services of others, especially at his local church and showing no interest or willingness to serve others. There are many 'Cliffords' around today and I pray you are not one of them. Always remember that you were not saved by your good works but by the finished work of Jesus through grace. However, God wants you to contribute to the well-being of others in the way you have been graced. He wants you to take from the lives of others and give something back in the way of service, thereby serving God.

Veronica said, "I don't think God will ever want to use me because I am not talented or gifted like other Christians." Dear Veronica, that's a lie from the devil. Every human being on earth has a unique ability which can be developed and put into use to benefit others. You were called into Christian ministry as soon as you became saved. 'Ministry is not only for apostles, prophets, evangelists, pastors and teacher. No. You can serve others with your gifts and talents. But first, the mind attitude of excuses and taking and taking but not being willing to give back has to be renewed with the word of God. Prayerfully read the passages of the scripture that teach that God is willing to use you. Read and meditate on them on a daily basis. Ask God to soften your heart and make you willing to be used by Him in any way to bless others for His glory.

QUESTIONS FOR REFLECTION

1. What motivated and still motivates Jesus to recruit more people into the harvest fields? (Harvest fields are the non-believers in Christ).

2. What are the requirements for being used by God to expand His kingdom or to serve others around you?

3. a) How would you encourage a Christian who feels that he or she is not adequate to be used by God? b) How would you talk to a Christian who seems reluctant to use their gifts or talents in your home group or even at Church?

NOTES

CHAPTER 30

LIVING DAILY AND MINISTERING UNDER OPEN HEAVEN

Heaven is a reality that is described so many times in the Bible, both in the Old and New Testament. The Hebrew word *shamayim* translated "heaven" is a plural noun that literally means "the heights." Among the heights is first the *atmospheric heaven* that covers the earth in form of clouds. **In six hundred year of Noah's life, on the seventeenth day of the second month . . . the floodgates of the heavens were opened. And rain fell on the earth for forty days and forty nights** (Genesis 7: 11&12). **He covers the sky with clouds; He supplies the earth with rain and makes grass to grow on the hills** (Psalm 147:8).

The second heaven is the *planetary heaven* were the stars, the moon, and the planets are located. **Then God said, let lights appear in the sky to separate the day from the night . . . God made two great lights—the larger one to govern the day, and the smaller one to govern the night. He also made the stars** (Genesis 1:14&16). **When I look at your heavens, the work of your fingers, the moon and the stars, which you have set in place, what is man that you are mindful of him, and the son of man that you care for him** (Psalm 8:3-4).

The third heaven is the home of God, His angels and all His saints. **I was caught up to the third heaven fourteen years ago. Whether I was in my body or out of my body, I don't know—only God knows . . . I was caught up to paradise and heard things so**

126

astounding that they cannot be expressed in words, things no
human is allowed to tell (2 Corinthians 12: 2&4). **Hearken to the
prayer of your servant and of your people Israel when they pray
in or toward this place. Hear in heaven, your dwelling place, and
when you hear, forgive** (1 King 8:30). **Pray therefore like this: Our
Father who is in heaven hallowed be your name** (Matthew 6:9).

This is the heaven from which Jesus came to earth and went
back to after His resurrection. This is the same heaven where your
born again spirit is right now seated with Jesus after its resurrection
from death in sin, to a spiritual life by the grace and mercy of God.
**And He raised us up together with Him and made us sit down
together (giving us joint seating with Him) in the heavenly
sphere (by virtue of our being) in Christ Jesus (the Messiah, the
Anointed One)** (Ephesians 2:6 AMP). **Since you have been raised
to new life with Christ, set your sights on the realities of heaven,
where Christ sits in the place of honour at God's right hand.
Think about the things of heaven, not the things of earth. For
you died to this life, and your real life is hidden with Christ in
God** (Colossians 3: 1-3). **And just as my father has granted me a
kingdom, I now grant you the right to eat and drink at my table
in my Kingdom. And you will sit on thrones, judging the twelve
tribes of Israel** (Luke 22:28-30).

May be only 20% of Spirit filled believers in Christ know that
heaven, the dwelling place of God was opened for them the moment
they became born again and it has remained open. This small
percentage of born again Christians live and operate under open
heaven made available by Jesus through His death and resurrection.
This 20% of believers in Christ know how to access boldly and enjoy
the open heaven by faith through unhindered communion with God
characterised by daily fresh revelations from the Holy Spirit on how
the will of God for them can be done here on earth as it is in heaven.
**Then as I look, I saw a door standing open in heaven, and the
same voice I heard before spoke to me like trumpet blast . . . said,
"come up here, and I will show you what must happen after this."**
(Revelation 4:1). **So then, since we have a great High Priest who
has entered heaven, Jesus the Son of God . . . . So let us come
boldly to the throne of our gracious God. There we will receive
His mercy, and we will find grace to help us when we need it**

(Hebrews 4:14&16). **Because of Christ and our faith in Him, we can now come boldly and confidently into God's presence** (Ephesians 3:12). **We have, then, my friends, complete freedom to go into the most Holy Place by means of the death of Jesus** (Hebrews 10:19 GNT). **Your kingdom come, your will be done on earth as it is in heaven** (Matthew 6:10).

Sadly, most Christians still live with the closed heaven mentality where they believe they need to perform in order for God to open up His heaven and may be give them tiny bits of blessings. If heaven is still closed, I don't think you will have a complete freedom to access it. But because of the blood of Jesus, heaven is wide open and you can enter freely and enjoy all that is in God through Jesus in your daily life according to your faith.

Everything you need to live a joyful, victorious and fulfilled life as the redeemed of the Lord is already within you because of Jesus who lives in you and who has also opened heaven for you so you can by faith constantly experience heaven while on earth as He did. **. . . the kingdom of God is within you** (Luke 17:21). **. . . Christ in you, the hope of glory** (Colossians 1:27 NIV). **. . . I tell you the truth; the Son can do nothing by Himself. He does only what He sees the Father doing. Whatever the Father does, the Son also does** (John 5:19). Everything you need to fulfil God's purpose in your life is already available for you in Christ by whom all things were created and for Him and whose joint heir you are. All you need is faith and wisdom to know how to live and minister under open heaven.

Josephina, a 20-year-old youth leader, originally from a non-Christian background said, "My understanding is that if I pray enough, give enough and serve enough at Church, then God will open the windows of heaven and give me some blessings." Josephina, you are already blessed in Christ as a believer. Ask the father in the name of Jesus and the Holy Spirit will release to you what is already yours. As a youth leader, you can through prayer freely enter into the throne of God and receive the healing which the stripes of Jesus has already provided for those you lead who need it.

You give or serve in appreciation of all that Jesus has already provided and not to get Him to do what He has already done. For many, praise and worship make it easy for their spirits to bring heaven to their daily human experience and ministry. To others it is quietness and meditation on Jesus, and to others, fasting. To many, fresh revelations like visions, dreams or word of knowledge or wisdom from the Holy Spirit about what God has for them and for the world around them increase their faith to receive. Find what works for you and keep to it. Remember, your heart attitude and burning desire should be to live and minister on earth under the heaven that is already open just as Jesus did.

QUESTIONS FOR REFLECTION

1. Which heaven is the home of God, His angels and His saints? Support answer with scriptures.
2. a) By what means as a believer in Christ was heaven opened to you for a free access? Explain with scriptures. b) What do you need to have in order to know how to live and minister under open heaven and what personally makes it easier for you to experience heaven on earth in different ways? c) Explain in your words the prayer-'your kingdom come, your will be done on earth as it is heaven.'
3. How would you counsel a believer in Christ who hasn't yet got it and is still struggling in different ways with closed heaven mentality?

NOTES

CHAPTER 31

HEALING ALL MANNER OF DISEASE

There was no limit to the type of sickness and disease that Jesus could heal because the Holy Spirit by whose power He ministered was greater than all sickness and disease that plagued people in His days on earth.

How God anointed Jesus of Nazareth with the Holy Spirit and power, and how He went around doing good and healing all who were under the power of the devil, because God was with Him (Acts 10:38). **Jesus went throughout Galilee, teaching in their Synagogues, proclaiming the good news of the kingdom, and healing every disease and sickness among the people** (Matthew 4:23). **Jesus went through all the towns and villages, teaching in their Synagogues, proclaiming the good news of the kingdom and healing every disease and sickness** (Matthew 9:35).

Today, many suffer from all kinds of sickness and Jesus can heal all through the Holy Spirit if the believers in Him can have the same trust He had on the Holy Spirit and allow Him to use them. Always remember that every Spirit filled believer has already got the power of God at work within them in one way or the other. The challenge is the willingness and availability of the people of God to be used by the Holy Spirit to release His healing power to the sick. **I tell you the truth, anyone who believes in me will do the same works I have done, and even greater works, because I am going to be with the father** (John 14:12). **Now to Him who is able to do immeasurably**

more than all we ask or imagine, according to His power that is at work within us (Ephesians 3:20).

If you are born again, you have the mind of Christ and so by His grace you can think like Him and judge situations the way He does, including healing the sick. You can choose to have the "All things are possible" mentality and step out boldly to heal all kinds of disease and sickness as Jesus commanded in **Matthew 10:1**, or you can choose to have the "What if it doesn't work" mentality and remain in your comfort zone till Jesus comes back. Note that there will be no pressure to perform when you remember that it is the Holy Spirit who does the healing miracle and not you. **The person with the Spirit makes judgments about all thing . . . who has known the mind of the Lord so as to instruct Him. But we have the mind of Christ** (1 Corinthians 2:15&16). **For God has not given us the Spirit of fear but of power, and of love, and of a sound mind** (2 Timothy 1:7 KJV). **Anything is possible if a person believes** (Mark 9:23). **Not by might nor by power, but by my Spirit, says the Lord Almighty** (Zechariah 4:6).

Most times, it is fear of failure that prevents Spirit filled Christians from exercising their faith in ministering healing to others, especially if the sickness is labelled "incurable" or "terminal."

Jonathan, a 27-year-old Bible College graduate confessed openly that he would rather not attempt to pray for a cancer sufferer than to pray and later see them die of the sickness. It is obvious that the underlying problem with Jonathan was fear of embarrassment if he failed to perform. The fear stemmed from doubt that Jesus could cure what is medically termed incurable disease. With much teaching, Jonathan came to understand that Jesus wanted and still wants to and is able to heal all manner of sickness as He did in the past. With His willingness, the healing of all kind of disease is possible. **What do you mean if I can? . . . Anything is possible if a person believes** (Mark 9:23). **You don't have enough faith . . . I tell you the truth, if you had faith even as small as a mustard seed, you could say to this mountain, 'move from here to there,' and it would move. Nothing would be impossible** (Matthew 17:18).

Even if the person you prayed for eventually died, that would not negate the truth that Jesus wanted them healed. When you are convinced deep within you that God loves everybody on earth and wants all sick people healed of any type of sickness, you are then in the state of mind where you can keep on believing for more healing and creative miracles in people's lives. Focus on what God is willing to do and is currently doing so you don't get discouraged and give up when things do not turn out the way you expect.

QUESTIONS FOR REFLECTON

1. Why could Jesus heal all types of sickness without any limit?
2. What could keep you from attempting to pray and believe for the healing of a person suffering from a life threatening illness?
3. a) What type of mentality can enable you to step out in faith to heal all kinds of disease and sickness as Jesus commanded in Matthew 10:1? b) What will protect you from the pressure to perform when you minister healing to the sick?

NOTES

CHAPTER 32

WHEN HEALING IS NOT
IMMEDIATELY MANIFESTED

Always remember that whether healing manifests immediately, gradually or not at all, it is still the will of God to heal the sick. Also bear in mind that God sent Jesus who purchased healing and forgiveness of sin for all mankind by His blood. Before His death, Jesus demonstrated God's will to heal people by healing all manner of disease and sickness. **News about Him spread as far as Syria, and people soon began bringing to Him all who were sick. And whatever their sickness or disease . . . He healed them all** (Matthew 4:24). **That evening many demon-possessed people were brought to Jesus. He cast out the evil spirits with a simple command, and He healed all the sick** (Matthew 8:16). **Everyone tried to touch Him, because healing power went out from Him, and He healed everyone** (Luke 6:19). **. . . and many people followed Him. He healed all the sick among them** (Mathew 12:15).

Jesus did not only demonstrate the will of God to heal all, He also authorised His disciples to heal everyone despite the type of disease or sickness. **Jesus called His disciples together and gave them authority to cast out evil spirits and to heal every kind of disease and sickness** (Matthew 10:1). **The apostles were performing many miraculous signs and wonders among the people . . . Crowds came from the villages around Jerusalem, bringing their sick and those possessed by evil spirits and they were all healed** (Acts 6:12&16).

There are many reasons why healing may not manifest immediately or why people are not healed. We have established from the scriptures that none of the reasons is because God does not want people healed. **. . . for I am the one who heals you** (Exodus 15:26b). **Dear friend, I pray that you enjoy good health and that all may go with you, even as your soul is getting along well** (3 John 2).

Don't blame yourself and get discouraged when you exercised your faith and ministered healing and nothing happened. Find out from the Holy Spirit the reason why healing did not manifest, but resolve to immediately move on whether or not you receive an explanation. Offer Jesus both the perplexity of not seeing the expected healing and the glory of the healing miracles He performs through you. None of them should be yours.

It is beyond the scope of this chapter to explore so many possible reasons why healing does not manifest immediately or manifest at all, but I will mention that sometimes healing is a process. **He looked at them and said, "Go show yourselves to the priests." And as they went, they were cleansed of their leprosy (Luke 17:14). Jesus took the blind man by the hand and led him out of the village. Then, spitting on the man's eyes, He laid His hand on him and asked, "Can you see anything now?" . . . he said, I see people . . . They look like trees walking around." Then Jesus placed His hands on the man's eyes again, and his eyes were opened . . . (Mark 8:23-25).**

I believe that doubt and unbelief are two of the main hindrances to healing. It will be hard for someone to receive or minister healing if they entertain the doubt that God wants mankind completely well or that God is able to cure what is humanly impossible. It's a state of mind and heart. It's about what dominates an atmosphere-faith or doubt? **And because of their unbelief, He couldn't do any miracles among them except to place His hands on a few sick people and heal them** (Mark 6:5). **But when you ask Him, be sure that your faith is in God alone. Do not waver, for a person with divided loyalty is as unsettled as a wave of the sea that is blown and tossed by the wind. Such people should not expect to receive anything from the Lord** (James 1:6&7).

Most times Jesus healed people out of His mercy and compassion with or without their faith. **Jesus saw the huge crowd as He stepped** from the boat, and He had compassion on them and healed their sick (Matthew 14:14). **Jesus felt sorry for them and touched their eyes. Instantly they could see. Then they followed Him** (Matthew 20:34). There were also other times when people received healing from Jesus as a result of their personal faith. **And He said to her, "Daughter, your faith has made you well. Go in peace. Your suffering is over."** (Mark 5:34). **And Jesus said to the man, "Stand up and go. Your faith has healed you."** (Luke 17:19)

Eugene said, "I've been a Christian all my life and I heard that God wants to heal me, but I have been battling with diabetes for years now despite all the prayers. I am thinking that may be God wants me to die with this sickness." I believe that Eugene's mindset represented the mindset of so many Christians who lack the knowledge of God's view on sickness and disease. I will encourage Eugene and others who think that God wants people to die with sickness to thoroughly search the scripture to establish the truth that Jesus respectively paid for their sickness and forgiveness with His blood that gushed out from His stripes and that which spilled when He was crucified on the cross. The day you received forgiveness through the new birth, you also received healing. I will encourage Eugene, if he received Jesus as Saviour and Lord to also receive Him as Healer by the same faith. By faith, expect your healing to manifest despite the symptoms. Look unto Jesus and listen to Him only and it shall be well with you in Jesus' name.

QUESTIONS FOR REFLECTION

1. How would you encourage someone you prayed for who didn't receive an instant healing? How would you handle it personally?
2. In your words, explain why healing may not manifest immediately or at all.
3. What will you tell a Christian person who has the mindset that God wants people to die with sickness?

NOTES

CHAPTER 33

DEALING WITH OTHER PEOPLE'S DOUBT

A ccording to the dictionary, doubt is a feeling of uncertainty or lack of conviction. In regards to divine healing, it means not being certain or convinced that God is willing or even able to heal a certain disease. Generally speaking, Christian life is a life of faith in God. **This Good News tells us how God makes us right in His sight. This is accomplished from start to finish by faith. As the Scriptures say, "It is through faith that a righteous person has life."** (Romans 1:17). **For we live by faith, not by sight** (2 Corinthians 5:7 NIV). **And without faith it is impossible to please God, because anyone who comes to him must believe that He exists and that He rewards those who earnestly seek him** (Hebrews 11:6).

There may be occasions when a person ministering healing to the sick has an unshakeable faith in God and believes deep within their heart that healing is already provided by God no matter the nature of the sickness, but they are surrounded by people who doubt God's ability or willingness to bring healing. In this type of situation, the best thing to do is to ignore, shun or avoid such people if possible. **When Jesus arrived at the official's home, He saw the noisy crowd and heard the funeral music. "Get out!" He told them. "The girl isn't dead; she's only asleep." But the crowd laughed at Him. And after the crowd was put outside, however, Jesus went in and took the girl by the hand, and she stood up** (Matthew 9:23-25). **Jesus took**

the blind man by the hand and led him out of the village. Then, spitting on the man's eyes, He laid His hands on Him and asked, "Can you see anything now?" . . . Then Jesus placed His hands on the man's eyes again, and his eyes were opened (Mark 8:23&25). Though it was not specifically stated that this event took place outside the village as a result of other people's possible doubt, it seemed most likely to be one of the reasons because previous verses indicated Jesus' disciples doubting that He could provide them with bread in the boat, when He had just fed four thousand people with seven loaves of bread and a few small fish (Mark 8:1-8). Jesus was only telling them to be careful with the Pharisees. (Mark 8:15).

At one time I shunned the doubt and resistance of a middle aged woman I was ministering to and released to her the creative miraculous power of the Holy Spirit based on the word of knowledge I received. A new vertebra was created and the hole at the woman's back was closed instantly to the glory of Jesus. At other times, I had ignored the doubt caused by familiarity and went ahead and released the healing power of the Holy Spirit according to the revelation knowledge I got and people received instant healings all to the glory of Jesus Christ.

On the other hand, a sick person may have the faith to receive healing but those around them may be full of doubt. The encouragement is to guard your heart and keep believing with thanks giving and confessing the word of God for healing. Your faith will see you through in Jesus' name. Amen. **Guard your heart above all else, for it determines the course of your life** (Proverbs 4:23). **For it is by believing in your heart that you are made right with God, and it is by confessing with your mouth that you are saved** (Romans 10:10). **Wait patiently for the Lord. Be brave and courageous. Yes, wait patiently** (Psalm 27:14). . . . **Because of your faith, it will happen** (Matthew 9:29). Child of God, build your faith and by God's grace release it in the atmosphere when you visit the sick, especially the one whose faith is weak. Look to the Holy Spirit to release the gift of faith to people around the sick person so that an impossible could become possible.

It takes the grace of God, courage and strong conviction of God's love and the finished work of Jesus for a believer with a life threatening illness to stand on the word of God and receive healing.

Pastor Debby was 45 years when she was diagnosed with breast cancer. Both her and her loved ones made a choice to stand on the word of God for her complete healing. According to her, she did everything possible to be on top of the situation through daily meditation and confession of the word of God. Throughout the period of chemotherapy, she, her family and close friends disregarded all the medical reports that had the potential to put fear and doubt in them and focused on Jesus. Glory to God that today Pastor Debby is cancer free and waxing strong in the work of the Lord.

QUESTIONS FOR REFLECTION

1. How would you define doubt in relation to divine healing?
2. How would you respond to those around you who seem to be doubting that the Holy Spirit will release healing to the person you are ministering to?
3. What do you do when you have faith to receive healing for yourself, but those around you are full of doubt?

NOTES

CHAPTER 34

HEALING THROUGH OTHER REMEDIES

People generally have natural faith in things and events based on experience. For example if you live in a place where there is constant supply of water, you have faith that whenever you turn on the tap, water will flow and not oil or any other liquid because it has always been that way. You have faith that the bed or chair will sustain your weight if they are in good condition. You have faith that after one Christmas there will be another one. There is no struggle to believe. It comes natural.

Our faith in God for healing based on Jesus' finished work should also be natural because His redemptive work is established and can be relied on just as you can rely on the Water Board for supply of no other liquid than water. Since it is His will to heal everyone, God can also extend his healing power to people through medicine.

You can choose to have a childlike faith in Jesus for your healing, or have the same faith for healing through other means by which He can also heal. The most important thing is to acknowledge that the healing you receive either by the supernatural release of God's healing power by the Holy Spirit or through medical intervention is as a result of the blood that gushed out of the wounds of Jesus Christ. Always remember that and return the glory to Him. **. . . What do you have that God hasn't given you? . . .** (1 Corinthians 4:7). **Whatever is good and perfect comes down to us from God our father, who created all the lights in the heavens. He never changes or** cast a shifting shadow (James 1:17). **But He was pierced for our transgressions, He was crushed for our iniquities; the punishment that brought us peace was on him, and by His wounds we are healed** (Isaiah 53:5).

Trust and glory should always be on the finished work of Jesus and His name and never on other remedies or Doctors and medical practitioners. **Trust in the Lord with all your heart; do not depend on your own understanding** (Proverb 3:5). **This is what the Lord says: "Cursed are those who put their trust in mere humans, who rely on humans strength and turn their hearts away from the Lord** (Jeremiah 17:5).

Jacob, a 26-year-old new Christian said, "I always feel guilty whenever I turn to the Doctor or the Chemist and depend totally on the prescription drugs instead of on God whenever I fall sick." I want to encourage you, Jacob not to feel guilty because God created Doctors and all the medical practitioners and gave them wisdom to use drugs made from natural but processed ingredients to cure various diseases. Always focus on Jesus irrespective of the way you are receiving or ministering healing. As a born again Christian, He is your Saviour and Healer. Give Him all the glory for the healing despite the method.

Though in the Bible times healing was ministered through other means apart from the direct release of God's supernatural healing power on the sick, it was still God at work. **. . . . This is what the Lord, the God of your ancestor David says:" I have heard your prayer and seen your tears. I will heal you . . ." Then Isaiah said, "Make an ointment from figs." So Hezekiah's servants spread the ointment over the boil, and Hezekiah recovered** (2 Kings 20:5&7). **So Naaman went down the Jordan River and dipped himself seven times, as the man of God had instructed him. And his skin became as healthy as the skin of a young child's, and he was healed** (2 Kings 5:14). **Then He spit on the ground, made mud with the saliva, and spread the mud over the blind man's eyes. He told him, "Go wash yourself in the pool of Siloam." So the man went and washed and came back seeing.** (John 9:6). **. . . . He put His fingers into the man's ears. Then, spitting on His own fingers, He touched the man's tongue. Looking up to heaven, He sighed and said, "Ephphatta," which means, "Be opened!" Instantly the man**

could hear perfectly and the tongue was freed so he could he could speak plainly (Mark 7:33-35).

Although God can heal through other remedies, I will encourage you to first acknowledge His willingness to manifest His supernatural healing power in your situation. In other words, though He can heal with medicine, start to practice looking unto Jesus to receive your healing from illnesses as minor as common cold, occasional headaches and the like. By so doing, you are building your faith on Jesus your Saviour and healer who has power over all kinds of disease and sickness. As for medicine, there is limit to what it can do in some situations labelled 'incurable,' but for Jesus, no sickness is incurable. Thank God for medicine, Doctors, Nurses and the like. As great as they are, they can fail in some health situations, but Jesus Christ will not fail if you totally put your trust in Him.

QUESTIONS FOR REFLECTION

1. How can you compare your natural faith with your faith in the finished work of Jesus in regards to healing?
2. What is the most important thing whether you receive divine healing or through medicine?
3. Why is it important for you to first look unto Jesus for divine healing, though He also heals through medicine?

NOTES

CHAPTER 35

HAVING A THANKFUL HEART NO MATTER WHAT

A web dictionary defines thankfulness as an attitude of heart from which you are aware of your blessings and show appreciation of them. I believe that a thankful attitude is developed and maintained from the knowledge that there is nothing one has that one has not received from God. . . . **What do you have that God hasn't given you?** (1 Corinthians 4:7). **Whatever is good and perfect comes down to us from God our Father, who created all the lights in heavens. He never changes or casts a shifting shadow** (James 1:17).

When it comes to Jesus' finished work in regards to our total healing and forgiveness, all believers in Christ owe it to God to daily maintain a thankful attitude to God and consciously advise our souls to praise and thank God no matter the situation. **Let all that I am praise the Lord; may I never forget the good things He does for me. He forgives all my sins and heals all my diseases** (Psalm 103:2&3). **Be thankful in all circumstances, for this is God's will for you who belong to Christ Jesus** (1 Thessalonians 5:18). Let your eyes remain fixed on Jesus even in adverse situations for He is working on your behalf. He is working in the ways you may not understand to show Himself strong in your weakness. . . . **My grace is all you need. My power works best in weakness** (2 Corinthians 12:9). **The eyes of the Lord search the whole earth in order to strengthen those whose hearts are fully committed to Him . . .** (2 Chronicles 16:9).

A believer in Christ can become grateful and full of praise despite their adverse situation when they receive a fresh revelation of Jesus, the extent of what He accomplished for them on the cross and what He plans to do for them.

This supernatural revelation or word of knowledge released by the Holy Spirit for that specific need is a great gift and a kind of fire that ignites the faith for the hour of need. It may come as a dream, a vision, and an inner witness or through the word of God. With this revelation, the Holy Spirit usually releases the gift of faith, a special kind of faith that will enable the person to believe the impossible. In other words, this believer knows with absolute certainty that they are already healed or that their need has already been met or that the person they are praying for or ministering to is already healed, no matter what. When this happens, the person can be full of joy and their heart is strengthened, looking forward to receiving what God has for them. They endure the hardship and with patience receive what is promised. . . . **Because of the joy awaiting Him, He endured the cross, disregarding its shame. Now He is seated in the place honour beside God's throne** (Hebrews 12:2). **I will certainly bless you, and I will multiply your descendants beyond number. Then Abraham waited patiently, and he received what God promised** (Hebrews 6:14&15).

Beatrice, a faith and Spirit filled woman of God in her 50s saw a vivid vision in her mind of how Jesus was bringing healing to her husband, Leo who was suffering from a severe digestive condition. Based on that supernatural revelation, Beatrice was instructed by the Holy Spirit to be and remain thankful for the revealed plan of God in regard to her husband's healing. She did. Beatrice chose to daily sing the praises of God, thanking Him in advance for Leo's healing. Even when Leo's condition seemed to be getting worse, Beatrice kept her eyes on Jesus at the exact place where she received the vision. The more she gazed at Jesus, the more supernatural revelations she received concerning the complete healing of her husband and the more thankful she became. Sooner than later, Leo was completely healed and waxing strong.

When you have a thankful heart toward God, your mind is stayed on Him and you are likely to be free of anxiety and enjoy His peace even in difficult times. **Do not be anxious about anything, but** in every situation, by prayer and petition, with thanksgiving, present your requests to God. And the peace of God which transcends all understanding will guard your hearts and your minds in Christ Jesus (Philippians 4:6&7). You will keep in perfect peace those whose minds are steadfast because they trust in you (Isaiah 26:3).

QUESTIONS FOR REFLECTION
1. How can you develop and maintain a thankful heart to God.
2. How can you become thankful and full of praise to God even in adverse situations?
3. Name some of the benefits you can enjoy when you have a thankful heart attitude toward God?

NOTES

CHAPTER 36

ALL GIFTS ARE FROM GOD.

G od is a generous giver. There are numerous scriptures that tell us that God is a giver and that everything you have has been given to you by Him and He is still giving. Take time then every moment of your life to give Him thanks for all you have through His generosity. **The Lord gives His people strength. The Lord blesses them with peace** (Psalm 29:11). **But thank God. He gives us victory over sin and death through our Lord Jesus Christ** (1 Corinthians 15:57). **For God loved the world so much that He gave His one and only, so that everyone who believes in Him will not perish but have eternal life** (John 3:16).

At new birth, God gives salvation to whoever shall believe, based on the finished work of Jesus Christ through the Holy Spirit who also baptises them into the body of Christ. **He saved us, not because of the righteous things we had done, but because of His mercy. He washed away our sins, giving us a new birth and new life through the Holy Spirit** (Titus 3:5). **Some of us are Jews, some are Gentiles, some are slaves, and some are free, but we have all been baptised into one body by one Spirit, and we all share the same Spirit** (1 Corinthians 12:13).

Jesus gave some people to the Church as gifts to equip the believers for the work of the ministry. **Now these are the gifts Christ gave to the Church: the apostles, the prophets, the evangelists, and the pastors and teachers. Their responsibility is to equip God's people to do His work and build up the Church, the body of Christ** (Ephesians 4:11&12).

Note that the Holy Spirit can lead anyone called into one of the ministry gifts to also operate in some or all the other offices. For example, an **apostle** called to plant Churches can also pastor those Churches at one time or the other before going to plant more as the Spirit leads.

A **prophet** serves as God's messenger, mouthpiece or spokesperson. He points to future events, reveals people's sins and advocates for repentance. Some prophets can also function in other ministry gifts as mentioned above.

An **evangelist** is called to preach the good news or the gospel to the unsaved, pointing them to Jesus and to the Church where he or she will also help them to grow and be prepared for their individual ministries. Remember that all believers in Christ are commissioned to preach the gospel.

A **pastor** is called to be the shepherd of the flock of God under his or her care. She or he has an oversight over the people of God and guides them. This servant of God gets the vision for the house of God, stewards the vision with his or her team, and moves the people of God forward by the vision through the Holy Spirit.

A **teacher** is called to accurately divide the written word of God as he or she invites the Holy Spirit to breathe upon the letters and make them alive and relevant to people's everyday needs.

The gift of the Holy Spirit

At Pentecost, Jesus fulfilled the promise He made to His disciples in Acts 1:8 and gave the believers the gift of the Holy Spirit (baptism in the Holy Spirit) to enable them be His witnesses. The same gift of the Holy Spirit is available to every believer in Christ today. **But you will receive power when the Holy Spirit comes upon you. And you will be my witnesses, telling people about me everywhere-in Jerusalem, throughout Judea, in Samaria, and to the ends of the earth** (Act 1:8). **On the day of Pentecost all believers were meeting together in one place. Suddenly, there was a sound from heaven like the roaring of a mighty windstorm, and filled the house where they were sitting. Then, what looked like flames or tongues of fire appeared and settled on each of them. And everyone present was filled with the Holy Spirit and began**

speaking in other languages as the Holy Spirit gave them this ability (Acts 2:1-4).

The fruit and gifts of the Holy Spirit

The Holy Spirit bears fruit in believers that will enable them grow into the image of Christ, gives them gifts that will motivate them into action. Motivation is a reason or reasons for acting or behaving in a particular way. The reason most believers allow the Holy Spirit to motivate them to use their spiritual gifts to benefit others is lest the grace be in vain in this day of salvation. **But the Holy Spirit produces this kind of fruit in our lives: love, joy, peace, patience, kindness, goodness, faithfulness, gentleness and self-control. There is no law against these things** (Galatians 5:22&23). **As God's co-workers, we urge you not to receive God's grace in vain. For He says, in the time of my favour I heard you, and in the day of salvation I helped you. I tell you, now is the time of God's favour, and now is the day of salvation** (2 Corinthians 6:1&2 NIV).

Motivational Spiritual gifts-

In His grace, God has given us different gifts for doing certain things well. So if God has given you the ability to prophesy, speak out with such faith as God has given you. If your gift is serving others, serve them well. If your gift is to encourage others, be encouraging. If it is giving, give generously. If God has given you leadership ability, take the responsibility seriously. And if you have a gift of showing kindness to others, do it gladly (Romans 12:6-8).

The Holy Spirit also manifests Himself and releases His nine gifts through the Church for the benefit of those who need those gifts at any given time as we shall see in the next chapter.

NOTES

CHAPTER 37

THE DEITY OF THE HOLY SPIRIT AND HIS NINE GIFTS

The Holy Spirit, as the third person in the Godhead shares equality with God the father and God the Son. **May the grace of our Lord Jesus Christ, and the love of God, and the fellowship of the Holy Spirit be with you all** (2 Corinthians 13:14). **Therefore, go and make disciples of all the nations, baptising them in the name of the father and the Son and the Holy Spirit** (Mathew 28:19).

In the person of the Holy Spirit, the Lord God is everywhere at the same time (Omnipresence). **I can never escape from your Spirit. I can never get away from your presence. If I go to heaven, you are there; if I go down to the grave, you are there** (Psalm 139:7&8). **Can anyone hide from me in a secret place? Am I not everywhere in all the heavens and earth? . . .** (Jeremiah 23:24).

The Holy Spirit, as God, knows all things (Omniscience). **But it was to us that God revealed these by His Spirit., for His Spirit searches out everything and shows us God's deep secrets** (1 Corinthians 2:10). **When the Spirit of truth comes, He will guide you into all truth. He will not speak of His own but will tell you what He heard. He will tell you about the future** (John 16:13).

The Holy Spirit being God is all powerful (Omnipotence). **. . . It is not by force nor by strength, but by my Spirit, says the Lord of heaven's Armies** (Zachariah 4:6). **My message and my preaching were not with wise and persuasive words, but with a demonstration of the Spirit's power, so that your faith might not**

rest on human wisdom, but on God's power (1 Corinthians 2:4&5). By His numerous gifts, the Holy Spirit demonstrates His power in and through the believers in Christ.

When you are baptised and filled with the Holy Spirit, you are filled with His power for ministry through His nine gifts which He can choose to manifest through you for those who are in need of them at any given time. **Now to each one is given the manifestation of the Spirit for the common good. For to one there is given the word of wisdom through the Spirit, and to another the word of knowledge according to the same Spirit; to another faith by the same Spirit, and to another gifts of healing by the one Spirit, and to another effecting of miracles, and to another prophecy, and to another the distinguishing of spirits, to another various kinds of tongues, and to another the interpretation of tongues** (1 Corinthians 12:7-10).

These nine gifts of the Holy Spirit are divided into three categories namely—Revelation gifts, vocal gifts and power gifts.

Revelation gifts
Word of wisdom
Word of knowledge
Distinguishing
of spirits

Vocal gifts
Prophecy
Tongues
Interpretation
of tongues

Power gifts
Gifts of healing
Working of miracles
Gift of faith

NOTES

CHAPTER 38

WORD OF WISDOM

Word of wisdom is a supernatural revelation of the Holy Spirit when the believer receives God's wisdom on what action to take in a given situation based on natural or supernatural knowledge. In other words, it is what God will want you to do about a particular situation you know of. If you look closely, you will see how the Holy Spirit used words of wisdom to instruct people on what to do in their particular situations in different ways such as:

By Inward witness of the Holy Spirit

Acts 16:6-10
Acts 20:22&23

Through the scriptures

Acts 1:15-23
Acts 15:13-21

By audible voice or by angel

1 Kings 19:12, and 15-18
Mark 9:7
Acts 8:26, 27 &29
Genesis 16:7-9

By vision and dream

Acts 18:9-10
Acts 16:9-10
Genesis 20:3-8&14
Matthew 1:20, 21&24

NOTES

CHAPTER 39

WORD OF KNOWLEDGE

The Bible talks much about wisdom, knowledge and understanding in relation to God and the affairs of mankind and they are considered great treasures from God. **Oh how great are God's riches and wisdom and knowledge. How impossible it is for us to understand His decisions and His ways** (Romans 11:33). . . . **I want them to have complete confidence that they understand God's mysterious plan, which is Christ Himself. In Him lie hidden the treasures of wisdom and knowledge** (Colossians 2:2&3). **By wisdom a house is built, and through understanding it is established; through knowledge its rooms are filled with rare and beautiful treasures** (Proverbs 24:3&4).

Word knowledge is a supernatural revelation by the Holy Spirit of some past or present facts about you, a person or a situation which cannot be known by human mind. It is just a small part of the whole picture which the Holy Spirit chooses to manifest for reasons such as prayer, protection, direction and the like. Note that in operating in the revelation and vocal gifts of the Holy Spirit, caution should be exercised to avoid announcing in public what God meant to be shared privately with the people concerned. Ask the Holy Spirit for the word of wisdom to know how to minister any word of knowledge which may come in various ways like:

Flow in thoughts as inner voice

John 4:16-18

John 11:11

Flow in pictures (Vision)

John 1:47&48
Hosea 12:10

As an audible voice

Acts 10:15
Ezekiel 43:6&7

As an angel

Acts 27:22-23
Luke 1:35&36

Generally speaking, the Holy Spirit in His sovereignty can manifest word of knowledge as flow of feelings, sudden impressions in your physical body. **Our God is in heaven; He does whatever pleases Him** (Psalm 115:3). **The Lord does whatever pleases Him throughout all heaven and earth, and on the seas and in their depths** (Psalm 135:6). The above scriptures remind us that we cannot box the Holy Spirit or restrict Him to known experiences. So you better watch out for His surprises. Sometimes it may be some physical discomfort in any part of your body that indicates the healing He wants to bring about in someone's body. Pay attention and respond immediately in prayer for further instruction. Obey at once as He leads.

NOTES

CHAPTER 40

DISTINGUISHING OF SPIRITS

Y ou are basically a spirit being. You have body and soul. As a born again Christian, your spirit was raised with Christ and seated with Him in the heavenly realms. That means you can now have spirit to Spirit interaction with God and know His deep things through the Holy Spirit. **Now may the God of peace make you holy in every way, and may your whole spirit and soul and body be kept blameless until our Lord Jesus Christ comes again** (1 Thessalonians 5:23). **For the word of God is alive and powerful. It is sharper than the sharpest two-edge sword, cutting between soul and spirit, between joint and marrow (Joints and marrow,** talking about your body) . . . . (Hebrews 4:12). **For He raised us from the dead along with Christ and seated us with Him in the heavenly realms because we are united with Christ.** (Ephesians 2:6). **But it was to us that God reveals these things by His Spirit, for His Spirit searches out everything and shows us God's deep secrets** (1 Corinthians 2:10).

Not only does the Holy Spirit show us the deep things of God, He, through the manifestation of the gift of distinguishing of spirits, can also show you the difference between Him, the human spirit, the spirit of the devil.

The gift of distinguishing of spirits is a supernatural ability to differentiate between the Spirit of God, the human spirit and demonic spirits. It is a God given ability to perceive or recognise the spirit behind a person, a situation, an action or a message.

In regards to the realm of God, the Holy Spirit can help you to know when it is the father talking to you, when Jesus is speaking, when He, the Holy Spirit is communicating what He has heard from the Father and the Son. You can even know when an angel is speaking to you. You develop this ability through an ongoing intimacy with the Holy Spirit. This and the other gifts of the Holy Spirit are His manifestations through whoever He chooses for the needs of another person. You don't need any special training to be used, except to be filled with the Holy Ghost and be willing and obedient.

The purpose of the gift of distinguishing of spirits is mainly to protect the church and prevent wrong spirits from influencing people. Having said this, one has to be careful not to discredit or despise out rightly the work of the Holy Spirit thereby grieving Him. Always ask Him to possess all of you so that the flesh will not get in the way when you operate in the gifts of the Holy Spirit.

Scriptural examples

Matthew 16:15-17
Matthew 16:22&23
Acts 16:16-18

NOTES

CHAPTER 41

GIFT OF PROPHECY

God always wants to talk to His children about His will on earth as it is in heaven. The gift of prophecy is different from the ministry gift of a prophet. The former is one of the manifestations of the Holy Spirit while the latter is one of the ministry gifts Jesus gave to the Church to equip the saints for the work of the ministry as seen previously in Ephesians 4:11. The utterances of a prophet are usually fore telling. In other words, they point to the future and what is in the heart of God. Please note that the New Testament prophet is speaking as the mouthpiece of Jesus, revealing the love of the father, His plans and purposes like Jesus did when He was on earth, and not like the prophets of old. **Long ago God spoke many times and in many ways to our ancestors through the prophets. And now in these final days, He has spoken to us through His Son** (Hebrews 1:1&2). **. . . For the essence of prophecy is to give a clear witness for Jesus** (Revelation 19:10). The prophet also reveals God's thoughts on sinful condition of a particular people group, warns gracefully and emphasises the need for repentance through the convincing power of the Holy Spirit.

The gift of prophecy is a spontaneous speaking forth as God's mouth piece under the direct supernatural influence of the Holy Spirit. The purpose of the gift of prophecy is to **edify** (to strengthen), to **exhort** (to encourage, to advice or to warn earnestly) and to **comfort** (to provide consolation with a great degree of tenderness). 1 Corinthians 14:3).

Scriptural examples

Luke 1:67-79
Mathew 20:17-19

The gift of prophecy is for today (The last days)

Acts 2:16-18
1 Corinthians 14:1&5

Prophecy is a small part of God's mind and not the whole picture

1 Corinthians 13:9
1 John 3:2

How prophecy is to be judged

By the scripture or (by Biblical principles for not everything is written in the Bible).

Hebrews 4:12
Isaiah 8:19&20

By the witness of the Holy Spirit within

1 John 2:27
1 Corinthians 2:15

By the confession of Jesus Christ

1 John 4: 1-3
Revelation 19:10

By its fruits of strength and liberty

1 Corinthians 14:3
Galatians 3:8

By the person's life

Matthew 7:15-20
Galatians 5:22&23

By fulfilment

Deuteronomy 18:21&22
Romans 15:12

To avoid disorderliness at a local church, the operation of the gift of prophecy and the other vocal gifts should be under the guidance of church leaders.

NOTES

CHAPTER 42

GIFT OF TONGUES AND INTERPRETATION OF TONGUES

The gift of tongue is supernatural ability given by the Holy Spirit to speak with a normal voice a language one does not know, to be interpreted in the body of Christ so that all may understand. This heavenly language is not learned by the speaker nor does it make any sense to them as they speak.

The gift of tongue as the manifestation of the Holy Spirit is different from the supernatural prayer or praise language given by the Holy Spirit on the day of Pentecost and when someone is baptised in the Holy Spirit. In the case of the gift of tongues, God speaks and man interprets to edify the Church. On the other hand, the tongues received at the baptism in the Holy Spirit is a supernatural private means of speaking mysteries to God and does not need to be interpreted because it is meant to edify the speaker and not the Church.

Scriptural examples of gift of tongues

1 Corinthians 12:10
1 Corinthians 14:5

Scriptural examples of tongues received at the baptism in the Holy Spirit

Acts 10:44-46
Acts 19:1-6

GIFT OF INTERPRETATION OF TONGUES

The gift of interpretation of tongues is a spontaneous God-given ability to interpret a message given in tongues for the understanding of the hearer. The knowledge of what is spoken in tongues is a direct manifestation of the Holy Spirit for the edification of the Church and has nothing to do with natural human knowledge and understanding.

Scriptural examples

1 Corinthians 12:10
1 Corinthians 14:13

NOTES

CHAPTER 43

GIFT OF FAITH

In the scriptures you find saving or general faith and the gift of faith. All are from God to man for personal relationship with Him and for the good of others. Saving or general faith is the initial faith by which you responded to God at your new birth, on which you also live as a believer in Christ. Jesus Christ is the giver of this faith through His word.

Scriptural examples of saving faith

Galatians 3:26
Ephesians 2:8

Jesus is the author

Hebrews 12:2
Romans 10:17
Romans 12:3
Romans 1:16

You live by this faith

Hebrews 10:38
2 Corinthians 5:6&7

This faith by which you live can grow through the word of God made alive by the Holy Spirit. It can also be tested and purified through trials. Without this faith it's impossible to please God. Jesus likes to find faith in you any time He comes. **. . . But when the Son of Man returns, how many will He find on earth who have faith?** (Luke 18:8) **. . . . Have faith in God** (Mark 11:22).

Gift of faith is a supernatural ability given by the Holy Spirit to believe for the naturally impossible. It is a manifestation of the Holy Spirit at a specific time and for a specific purpose. This type of faith is not the general faith which believes God for breakthrough, but a special faith released by the Holy Spirit where you just know that God wants to do a specific thing. In other words, the gift of faith is solely dependent on the revelation knowledge of the will of God which can come as dreams, visions, inner voice, impressions on the physical body or by the written word of God made alive for a particular need. Just as the general faith comes by hearing the word of God, so also does gift of faith come by knowing the will of God to meet a need.

Scriptural examples of gift of faith (In Jesus and the apostles)

Matthew 8:1-3
John 9:1-3&6-7
Acts 3:1-7
Acts 20:7-12

Note that the gift of faith often works alongside other gifts. For example in the above story as seen in John 9, Jesus had a word of knowledge that the child's blindness was not as a result of sin, but for the glory of God. He received a word of wisdom to heal with mud made out of His saliva.

NOTES

Chapter 44

GIFTS OF HEALING

Gifts of healing are the supernatural ability given by the Holy Spirit to impart His healing power into people who need healing at specific times. They are called gifts of healing for some reasons, two of which are: 1) **Some of the others gifts are often directly manifested when we minister healing to people.** 2) **There are many ways to impart healing.** For example, you may receive a word of knowledge about the root cause of someone's condition and also receive the gift of distinguishing of spirit if a spirit is behind it. The Holy Spirit can at the same time release word of wisdom to you on how to minister healing. With this, the gift of faith becomes actively involved; causing the healing or instant miraculous power of the Holy Spirit to be released to the person needing the miracle.

Scriptural examples of other gifts being directly involved in healing

Matthew 9:1-7
Luke 18:35-43
Acts 14:8-10
Acts 9:32-33

Scriptural examples of other ways by which healing can be ministered

Healing can be instantaneous

Matthew 8:3

Mark 1:29-31
Acts 3:1-8
Acts 9:32-35

Healing can be gradual

Mark 8:22-26
Luke 17:11-14

Healing by laying on of hands

Mark 1:40-41
Mark 7:31-35
Acts 28:8
Mark 16:16-18

Healing by anointing with oil

Mark 6:13
James 5:14

Healing by touch of garment or shadow or garment

Mark 6:56
Acts 5:15-16

Healing through handkerchiefs or aprons

Acts 19:11-12

Healing is based on faith and also by God's mercy and compassion

Healing is based by faith

Luke 18:35-43
Mark 5:25-34

Healing is based on God's mercy and compassion

Matthew 14:14
Mark 1:40-42
Matthew 15:29-31

Jesus did many other things that were not recorded

John 20:30
John 21:25

If you believe you can do what Jesus did and even more

John 14:12

Jesus commissioned you
Matthew 10:1
Mark 16:15-18
Matthew 28:18-20

You are the righteous and so be bold as lions (Proverbs 28:1) and preach the gospel, cast out demons and heal all kinds of disease and sickness in the name of Jesus by the power of the Holy Spirit because Jesus has authorised you.

NOTES

CHAPTER 45

GIFT OF WORKING OF MIRACLES

I n the New Testament, the word 'miracle' is from the Greek word dunamis. It portrays God's power or energy. From dunamis we have the English word 'dynamite.' Dynamite is an explosive material made with clay or powdered shells used for blasting or demolishing buildings or mining.

In the spiritual realm, this is a picture of the type of power a believer in Christ possesses through the Holy Spirit, which when released in different areas of human life establishes the kingdom of God to a certain degree if not entirely. **For I am not ashamed of this Good News about Christ. It is the power of God at work, saving everyone who believes-the Jew first and also the Gentile** (Romans 1:16). **But if I am casting out demons by the power of God, then the kingdom of God has arrived among you** (Luke 11:20).

Gift of working of miracle is a spontaneous and supernatural demonstration of the power of the Holy Spirit in human affairs which cannot be explained on any natural basis.

Miracles are significant part of the Bible. Jesus demonstrated the miraculous power of the Holy Spirit in His days on earth and so did the apostles. As it was in the days of Jesus and those of the apostles, so also it is meant to be in our days because the same Holy Spirit has been given to every believer.

Scriptural examples of miracles by Jesus

John 2:1-11
John 4:46-54

Scriptural examples of miracles by the disciples

Acts 8:4-8
Acts 19:11-12

For believers in Christ today

Mark 16:15-20
Matthew 10:1
John 14:12

How to operate daily in these nine gifts

Many of us Christians identify the Holy Spirit with His power, His gifts, His fruit and all He does for us. Some even identify Him with His symbols like fire, wind, water, oil and dove without knowing or remembering that the Holy Spirit is a distinct person in the Godhead who has personality. Personality refers to one's unique way of thinking, feeling and acting. It refers to one's intelligence, feeling and will. Always bear in mind that God the Father, God the Son and God the Holy Spirit are One God. They have the same nature and character but express them in distinct ways. It is a mystery, though.

The starting point in the daily operation of the gifts is to seek to know the Holy Spirit at an intimate level. As God, your maker, He knows everything about you and it remains for you to know Him. Remember that He is a person. He has will, emotions and possesses intelligence. Just think about it, though you are a human being, you have a unique personality. It is the same with the Holy Spirit. Though He is God, He has His own personality distinct and separated from that of the Father and the Son.

As He communed with the people in the Bible days and still does with the saints of God today, so does the Holy Spirit want to fellowship and speak to you when you seek intimacy with Him. As a unique person, the Holy Spirit wills to talk to you in unique ways even when it comes to releasing His gifts through you. You can only know His ways and hear His voice when you draw closer to Him in fellowship. **May the grace of the Lord Jesus Christ, the love of God, and the fellowship of the Holy Spirit be with you all** (2 Corinthians 13:14). **The Holy Spirit said to Philip, "Go over and walk along beside the carriage." Philip ran over and heard the man reading from the prophet Isaiah . . .** (Act 8:29&30). **The Holy Spirit told me to go with them and not to worry that they were Gentiles. These six brothers here accompanied me, and we soon entered the home of the man who had sent for us** (Acts 11:13).

An ongoing intimate relationship with the Holy Spirit and being daily filled with Him will likely cause you to hunger and be more desperate for Him to possess you more and more. He is the one who actually creates that hunger as you get closer to Him. The Holy Spirit loves your friendship and He delights to release His gifts through you as you eagerly desire them for the good of others so that Jesus will be glorified. **Anyone who is thirsty may God to me. Anyone who believes in me may come and drink. For the scriptures declare, 'Rivers of living water will flow from his heart.' When He said "Living water" He was speaking of the Spirit . . .** (John 7:38&39). **. . . Be filled with the Holy Spirit** (Ephesians 4:18). **After this prayer, the meeting place shook, and they were filled with the Holy Spirit. Then they preached the word of God with boldness** (Acts 4:31). **Follow the way of love and eagerly desire gifts of the Spirit, especially to prophecy** (1 Corinthians 14:1 NIV). **So it is with you. Since you are eager for gifts of the Spirit, try to excel in those that build up the Church** (1Corinthians 14:12).

With an ongoing intimate relationship with the Holy Spirit, you are in a good position to talk to Him freely about anything that may prevent you from operating in any of His gifts. Tell Him to help you deal with it, no matter what. You can also share the joy of your breakthroughs with Him as He releases His gifts through you and helps you to immediately give the glory to Jesus. In this intimate relationship with the Holy Spirit, you can also share your feeling of disappointment when things don't go as you wish, like when someone you prayed for died. He will comfort and give you courage to keep ministering.

Earnestly desire to operate daily in those gifts of the Holy Spirit that will bring to people and will demonstrate God's power to the world that does not acknowledge Him. You can only get as much as you are hungry for. Be desperate for word of knowledge, gift of faith, and working of miracles and gifts of healing through which the Holy Spirit can demonstrate His power and cause unbelievers to surrender to Jesus as you preach the gospel. In fact desire to operate in all of the gifts of the Holy Spirit for the good of others, for your own good and to the glory of Jesus.

Note that it is very important that our earnest desire for the gifts of the Holy Spirit is motivated by love for God and for humanity. Love is what you choose to do or give and not what you say or feel. You cannot love without giving. **Dear children, let's not merely say that we love each other; let us show the truth by our actions** (1John 3:18). **For God so loved the world that He gave His one and only Son, that everyone who believes in Him will not perish but have eternal life** (John 3:16).

How to operate in the miraculous

In almost all cases, God requires a human agent to carry out His miraculous deeds. This does not mean He cannot do it all alone, but He chose to work with mankind for His glory and for the good of the instrument used.

Miracles are based on the will of God and so He wants to communicate to you His mind or will concerning a situation.

1) Know His will

Scriptural examples

Ezekiel 37:1-6
Exodus 14:16
John 5:19

2) Believe what God reveals

Scriptural examples

Genesis 15:5-6
Hebrews 11:7

3) Speak like God (Not letter, but the exact word for the situation given by the Holy Spirit, for the letter kills. 2 Corinthian 3:6).

Scriptural examples

Psalm 33:6
Romans 4:17

**4). Issue faith command based on revelation knowledge only.
Scriptural examples**

John 11:43-44
John 5:8-9
Acts 3:6-7

Apart from the outward demonstration of the miraculous power of God, the greatest miracle of all is the salvation of human spirit from the power of sin through the Gospel or the Good News of Jesus Christ. This is followed by the inner miraculous deeds of the Holy Spirit that transform the believer in Christ from glory to glory. No one can do these inner works except the Holy Spirit.

Scriptural examples

Romans 1:16
Ephesians 3:20
2 Corinthians 3:16&18

Appeal for the greatest miracle—the salvation of your spirit from sin.

If you are not sure whether or not you are saved, it's most likely that you are not or that you've backslidden and gone the opposite way. Either way, God wants you back. He loves you too much to let go. It's not the good stuff you do or the church services you attend that will save you from the power of sin. It is by the grace of God through the finished work of Jesus Christ on the cross.

The only way to access this grace and find forgiveness is by the new birth of your spirit as Jesus made clear in **John 3:3**. I appeal to you in the name of Jesus to surrender and have this wonderful miracle. If you are ready, you can pray this simple prayer-

God in heaven I am sorry for my sins. I sincerely ask you to forgive me. I choose to receive Jesus Christ as my Saviour, Healer and Lord. Jesus Christ please come into my heart as my Saviour, my Healer and my Lord. Wash my sins away with your blood and baptise me in the Holy Spirit. I believe in my heart and I call you my Lord. Thank you Lord Jesus. I am saved.

You are welcome or welcome back to the family of God. Get yourself a New Testament Bible and read it on a daily basis. Start with the gospel of John so you get a clear picture of Jesus' love for you. Find a Bible based Church and attend regularly. Talk to God in prayer in the name of Jesus. Befriend the Holy Spirit and seek intimacy with Him for He's the one that reveals Jesus and helps you to live a victorious and joyful Christian life where backsliding is not an option. Live a day at a time in Christ and you will mature as a mighty man or woman of God in Jesus' name. Amen.

NOTES

CHAPTER 46

A CALL FOR TESTIMONY

According to Wikipedia, testimony is a legal form of evidence obtained under oath from a witness who makes a solemn statement or declaration about an event or experience. Online Dictionary defines a witness as one who can give a firsthand account of something seen, heard or experienced.

Although there are many gods in this world, the triune God—God the Father, God the Son and God the Holy Spirit is the only true and living God who created the heaven and the earth and everything that is in them. He counts on you as well as other believers in Him to bear Him witness to the world around you of His sovereignty, His love, His great miracles and all that He is as you personally experience Him. **But you are my witnesses, O Israel . . . you are my servant. You have been chosen to know me, believe in me and understand that I alone am God. There is no other God—there never has been, and there never will be.** (Isaiah 43:10). **Give thanks to the Lord and proclaim His greatness. Let the whole world know what He has done. . . . Tell everyone about His wonderful deeds** (Psalm 105:1&2). **Has the Lord redeemed you? Then speak out. Tell others He has redeemed you from your enemies** (Psalm 107:2). **We cannot stop telling about everything we have seen and heard** (Acts 4:20).

THE POWER OF YOUR TESTIMONY

1. Your testimony glorifies Jesus
   Your Christian life is for the glory of Jesus and so the Holy
   Spirit delights in working in, through and for you as an
   opportunity to bring glory to Jesus. It is then left to you to
   testify and glorify Jesus. **After that visit, I went north into
   the provinces of Syria and Cilicia. And still the Christians in
   the Churches in Judea didn't know me personally. All they
   knew was that people were saying, "The one who used to
   persecute us is now preaching the very faith He tried to
   destroy." And they praise God because of me** (Galatia 1:21-
   24). **The woman left her water Jar beside the well and ran
   back to the village telling everyone, "come and see a man
   who told me everything I ever did. Could He possibly be
   the Messiah?"** (John 4:28&29).

2. Your testimony draws people to Christ and causes them to
   believe and receive blessings from God.
   **Many Samaritans from the village believed in Jesus
   because the woman said," He told me everything I ever
   did** (John 4:39). **Peter's words pierced their hearts, and
   they said to him and to the other apostles, "Brothers what
   should we do?" . . . Those who believed what Peter said
   were baptised and added to the Church that day about
   3,000 in all** (Acts 2: 37&41).

3. The word of God that backs your testimony overcomes the
   devil.
   **And they overcame him by the blood of the Lamb and
   by the word of their testimony . . .** (Revelation 12:11). **It is
   written, 'Man shall not live by bread alone, but by every
   word that proceeds from the mouth of God** (Matthew 4:4)
   **It is written again, "You shall not tempt the Lord your
   God."** (Matthew 4:7). **. . . Then the devil left, and behold,
   angels came and ministered to Him** (Matthew 4:11).

HOW TO GIVE YOUR TESTIMONY

1. Invite the Holy Spirit to help you glorify Jesus.
2. Be joyful and enthusiastic as you tell your story in order to arouse people's interest. Always maintain eye contact as much as you can so as to engage the people.
3. Focus on Jesus and avoid being overly impressed by what the devil did before your breakthrough. Use the word of God for that season as you briefly state the challenge.
4. Also state briefly how you received the breakthrough, using the word of God that sustained and brought you the victory. This is how you overcome the devil.
5. Share joyfully how life is different for you as a result of God's intervention and give all the glory to Jesus.

QUESTIONS FOR REFLECTION

1. Describe in your words what you understand by 'testimony' and 'witness' in regards to your relationship with God.
2. Why is your testimony of God important?
3. According to the author, how are you to share your testimony?

NOTES

CHAPTER 47

CONCLUSION

Man sinned and satan brought sickness to humanity, but God wants all people healed and saved, hence Jesus' suffering for humanity. Divine healing is part of salvation and should be received, ministered and preached as such so that people will understand and receive divine healing with same faith by which they receive the salvation of their spirits.

Despite what you do for a living, you as a believer together with other believers in Him, have been commissioned by Jesus to preach the gospel, heal the sick, raise the dead, cast out demons and cleanse the leper. It is not a suggestion, but a command that can only be obeyed by the help and empowerment of the Holy Spirit as you become more intimate with Him. When you believe that by the stripes of Jesus you are already healed and that you can also do the works that Jesus did and even more, the Holy Spirit can then help you to receive and minister divine healing by faith despite any contrary physical condition or report.

Apart from faith, God can also release His healing power to the sick out of His mercy and compassion. He can also heal through medicine, but always remember that He is the healer and all the glory should be His. However, there are some physical conditions which may be beyond the healing ability of the medical practitioners, which only God the Holy Spirit can provide healing for. For this reason, you are encouraged to begin in time to exercise your faith in Christ for divine healing so your heart can receive the gift of faith from the Holy Spirit where there is need to believe for the impossible in a critical health condition.

You are the temple of God, and so common-sense demands that you look after God's house by keeping it healthy and fit. Always remember that you are a vessel that God made for His use to heal the sick and bring the loss back home, so look after your spirit, soul and body.

NOTES